T0227390

Anemia and Heart Failure

Guest Editors

ANIL K. AGARWAL, MD, FACP, FASN
STUART D. KATZ, MD
AJAY K. SINGH, MB, FRCP

HEART FAILURE CLINICS

www.heartfailure.theclinics.com

Consulting Editors
RAGAVENDRA R. BALIGA, MD, MBA
JAMES B. YOUNG, MD

Founding Editor
JAGAT NARULA, MD, PhD

July 2010 • Volume 6 • Number 3

SAUNDERS an imprint of ELSEVIER, Inc.

W.B. SAUNDERS COMPANY
A Division of Elsevier Inc.

1600 John F. Kennedy Boulevard • Suite 1800 • Philadelphia, Pennsylvania 19103-2899

http://www.theclinics.com

HEART FAILURE CLINICS Volume 6, Number 3
July 2010 ISSN 1551-7136, ISBN-13: 978-1-4377-2456-1

Editor: Barbara Cohen-Kligerman

© 2010 Elsevier Inc. All rights reserved.

This journal and the individual contributions contained in it are protected under copyright by Elsevier, and the following terms and conditions apply to their use:

Photocopying

Single photocopies of single articles may be made for personal use as allowed by national copyright laws. Permission of the Publisher and payment of a fee is required for all other photocopying, including multiple or systematic copying, copying for advertising or promotional purposes, resale, and all forms of document delivery. Special rates are available for educational institutions that wish to make photocopies for non-profit educational classroom use. For information on how to seek permission visit www.elsevier.com/permissions or call: (+44) 1865 843830 (UK)/(+1) 215 239 3804 (USA).

Derivative Works

Subscribers may reproduce tables of contents or prepare lists of articles including abstracts for internal circulation within their institutions. Permission of the Publisher is required for resale or distribution outside the institution. Permission of the Publisher is required for all other derivative works, including compilations and translations (please consult www.elsevier.com/permissions).

Electronic Storage or Usage

Permission of the Publisher is required to store or use electronically any material contained in this journal, including any article or part of an article (please consult www.elsevier.com/permissions). Except as outlined above, no part of this publication may be reproduced, stored in a retrieval system or transmitted in any form or by any means, electronic, mechanical, photocopying, recording or otherwise, without prior written permission of the Publisher.

Notice

No responsibility is assumed by the Publisher for any injury and/or damage to persons or property as a matter of products liability, negligence or otherwise, or from any use or operation of any methods, products, instructions or ideas contained in the material herein. Because of rapid advances in the medical sciences, in particular, independent verification of diagnoses and drug dosages should be made.

Although all advertising material is expected to conform to ethical (medical) standards, inclusion in this publication does not constitute a guarantee or endorsement of the quality or value of such product or of the claims made of it by its manufacturer.

Heart Failure Clinics (ISSN 1551-7136) is published quarterly by Elsevier Inc., 360 Park Avenue South, New York, NY 10010-1710. Months of publication are January, April, July, and October. Business and editorial offices: 1600 John F. Kennedy Boulevard, Suite 1800, Philadelphia, PA 19103-2899. Periodicals postage paid at New York, NY, and additional mailing offices. Subscription prices are USD 193.00 per year for US individuals, USD 326.00 per year for US institutions, USD 67.00 per year for US students and residents, USD 232.00 per year for Canadian individuals, USD 374.00 per year for Canadian institutions, USD 247.00 per year for international individuals, USD 374.00 per year for international institutions, and USD 85.00 per year for Canadian and foreign students/residents. To receive student and resident rate, orders must be accompanied by name of affiliated institution, date of term, and the *signature* of program/residency coordinator on institution letterhead. Orders will be billed at individual rate until proof of status is received. Foreign air speed delivery is included in all *Clinics* subscription prices. All prices are subject to change without notice. **POSTMASTER:** Send address changes to *Heart Failure Clinics*, Elsevier Health Sciences Division, Subscription Customer Service, 3251 Riverport Lane, Maryland Heights, MO 63043. **Customer Service: 1-800-654-2452 (US and Canada). From outside of the US and Canada, call 314-447-8871. Fax: 314-447-8029. For print support, e-mail: JournalsCustomerService-usa@elsevier.com. For online support, e-mail: JournalsOnlineSupport-usa@elsevier.com.**

Reprints. For copies of 100 or more of articles in this publication, please contact the Commercial Reprints Department, Elsevier Inc., 360 Park Avenue South, New York, NY 10010-1710. Tel.: 212-633-3812; Fax: 212-462-1935; E-mail: reprints@elsevier.com.

Heart Failure Clinics is covered in *MEDLINE/PubMed (Index Medicus)*.

Cover artwork courtesy of Umberto M. Jezek.

Printed and bound by CPI Group (UK) Ltd, Croydon, CR0 4YY

Transferred to Digital Print 2011

Contributors

CONSULTING EDITORS

RAGAVENDRA R. BALIGA, MD, MBA
Professor of Internal Medicine,
Vice Chief and Assistant Division
Director, Division of Cardiovascular
Medicine, The Ohio State University,
Columbus, Ohio

JAMES B. YOUNG, MD
Professor of Medicine and Executive Dean,
Cleveland Clinic Lerner College of Medicine;
George and Linda Kaufman Chair, Chairman,
Endocrinology and Metabolism Institute,
Cleveland Clinic, Cleveland, Ohio

GUEST EDITORS

ANIL K. AGARWAL, MD, FACP, FASN
Professor of Medicine, Director of
Interventional Nephrology, Division of
Nephrology, The Ohio State University,
Columbus, Ohio

STUART D. KATZ, MD
Professor of Medicine, Director of Heart
Failure, Division of Cardiology, School of

Medicine, New York University Langone
Medical Center, New York, New York

AJAY K. SINGH, MB, FRCP(UK)
Physician, Renal Division, Brigham and
Women's Hospital, Harvard Medical School,
Boston, Massachusetts

AUTHORS

ANIL K. AGARWAL, MD, FACP, FASN
Professor of Medicine, Director of
Interventional Nephrology, Division of
Nephrology, The Ohio State University,
Columbus, Ohio

**INDER S. ANAND, MD, FACC, FRCP,
DPhil (Oxon)**
Director, Heart Failure Program, Veterans
Affairs Medical Center; Professor of Medicine,
University of Minnesota Medical School,
Minneapolis, Minnesota

STEFAN D. ANKER, MD, PhD
Department of Cardiology, Charite Medical
School, Berlin, Germany; Centre for Clinical
and Basic Research, IRCCS San Raffaele
Roma, Rome, Italy

SALMAN ARAIN, MD
Assistant Professor of Medicine, Tulane Heart
and Vascular Institute, Tulane University
School of Medicine, New Orleans, Louisiana

PHILIPP ATTANASIO, MD
Department of Cardiology, Charite Medical
School, Berlin, Germany

RUDOLF A. DE BOER, MD, PhD
Cardiologist, Department of Cardiology,
University Medical Center Groningen,
University of Groningen, Groningen,
The Netherlands

EWA A. JANKOWSKA, MD, PhD, FESC
Department of Heart Diseases, Wroclaw
Medical University; Centre of Heart Diseases,
Military Hospital, Wroclaw, Poland

QURAT-UL-AIN JELANI, MD
The Leon H. Charney Division of Cardiology,
New York University School of Medicine,
New York, New York

STUART D. KATZ, MD
Professor of Medicine, Director of Heart
Failure, Division of Cardiology, School of
Medicine, New York University Langone
Medical Center, New York, New York

MIKHAIL KOSIBOROD, MD
Associate Professor, Saint Luke's
Mid-America Heart Institute and University
of Missouri-Kansas City School
of Medicine, Kansas City, Missouri

THIERRY H. LE JEMTEL, MD
Professor of Medicine, Tulane Heart and
Vascular Institute, Tulane University School of
Medicine, New Orleans, Louisiana

ELDRIN F. LEWIS, MD, MPH
Assistant Professor of Medicine,
Cardiovascular Division, Department of
Medicine, Brigham and Women's Hospital,
Boston, Massachusetts

ERIK LIPŠIC, MD, PhD
Cardiology Resident, Department of
Cardiology, University Medical Center
Groningen, University of Groningen,
Groningen, The Netherlands

ROBERT J. MENTZ, MD
Medical Resident, Department of Internal
Medicine, Brigham and Women's Hospital,
Boston, Massachusetts

TEJAS V. PATEL, MD
Fellow, Renal Division, Brigham and Women's
Hospital, Boston, Massachusetts

PIOTR PONIKOWSKI, MD, PhD, FESC
Department of Heart Diseases, Wroclaw
Medical University; Centre of Heart Diseases,
Military Hospital, Wroclaw, Poland

WILLEM-PETER T. RUIFROK, MD
Research Physician, Department of
Experimental Cardiology, University Medical
Center Groningen, University of Groningen,
Groningen, The Netherlands

ADAM C. SALISBURY, MD
Saint Luke's Mid-America Heart Institute and
University of Missouri-Kansas City School of
Medicine, Kansas City, Missouri

AJAY K. SINGH, MB, FRCP(UK)
Physician, Renal Division, Brigham and
Women's Hospital, Harvard Medical School,
Boston, Massachusetts

RICHARD K. SPENCE, MD, MHA, FACS
Medical Officer, Haemonetics, Braintree,
Massachusetts; Former Professor of Surgery,
Robert Wood Johnson School of Medicine,
University of Medicine and Dentistry of New
Jersey, Camden, New Jersey

W.H. WILSON TANG, MD
Section of Heart Failure and Cardiac
Transplantation Medicine, Heart and Vascular
Institute, Cleveland Clinic, Cleveland, Ohio

WIEK H. VAN GILST, PhD
Professor of Cardiovascular and Clinical
Pharmacology, Department of Experimental
Cardiology, University Medical Center
Groningen, University of Groningen,
Groningen, The Netherlands

DIRK J. VAN VELDHUISEN, MD, PhD
Professor of Cardiology, Department of
Cardiology, University Medical Center
Groningen, University of Groningen,
Groningen, The Netherlands

P.S. DANIEL YEO, MBBS, MRCP(UK)
Department of Cardiovascular Medicine, Tan
Tock Seng Hospital, Republic of Singapore

Contents

Editorial xi

Ragavendra R. Baliga and James B. Young

Preface xvii

Anil K. Agarwal, Stuart Katz, and Ajay K. Singh

Epidemiology of Anemia in Heart Failure 271

W.H. Wilson Tang and P.S. Daniel Yeo

Anemia is being increasingly recognized as an important comorbidity in patients with heart failure. Despite wide variations in defining anemia, approximately one-fifth to one-third of patients with heart failure may experience anemia at a given time. The prevalence may increase to more than half of patients in the setting of severe heart failure, and it may differ with different settings. Meanwhile, up to a fifth of patients may experience new-onset anemia, even though most cases may resolve over time. Different factors contribute to the development of anemia, including increasing age, renal insufficiency, hemodilution, chronic inflammation, and increasing heart failure disease severity.

Pathophysiology of Anemia in Heart Failure 279

Inder S. Anand

Renal dysfunction and neurohormonal and proinflammatory cytokine activation appear to contribute to anemia of chronic disease in most patients, resulting in inappropriate erythropoietin production and defective iron utilization. Under normal conditions, reduced tissue oxygenation caused by chronic anemia results in non-hemodynamic and hemodynamic compensatory responses to enhance oxygen carrying capacity. Erythropoiesis is the predominant non-hemodynamic response to hypoxia, but because erythropoiesis is defective in heart failure, hemodynamic mechanisms may predominate in chronic severe anemia. Hemodynamic responses are complex and involve a vasodilation-mediated high-output state with neurohormonal activation. The high output state initially helps to increase oxygen transport. However, the hemodynamic and neurohormonal alterations could potentially have deleterious long-term consequences and may contribute to anemia's role as an independent risk factor for adverse outcomes.

Mediators of Anemia in Chronic Heart Failure 289

Thierry H. Le Jemtel and Salman Arain

Anemia is highly prevalent in patients with chronic heart failure (CHF) and is associated with poor clinical outcome. Increased prevalence of anemia in CHF has been linked to advanced age, female gender, renal function impairment, severity of symptoms, and clinical settings. Overall, the anemia of CHF shares many common features with the anemia of chronic disease. Both impaired iron metabolism and inflammatory stress appear to be the key mediators of the anemia of CHF.

Molecular Changes in Myocardium in the Course of Anemia or Iron Deficiency   295

Ewa A. Jankowska and Piotr Ponikowski

Chronic untreated anemia or iron deficiency (ID) can result in an increased cardiac output, chronic sympathetic activation, left ventricular hypertrophy, and left ventricular dilation, leading to symptomatic chronic heart failure (CHF). Only in the past decade has there been an increase in interest in anemia and ID occurring in the course of CHF. The pharmacologic support in erythropoietin signaling or the correction in iron metabolism may activate molecular pathways that can protect the heart and prevent myocardial remodeling, and hence become a novel therapeutic approach in patients with CHF. Most of the data come from experimental models. Further studies, in particular performed in clinical settings, are warranted.

Treatment with Iron of Patients with Heart Failure With and Without Anemia   305

Qurat-ul-ain Jelani, Philipp Attanasio, Stuart D. Katz, and Stefan D. Anker

Iron deficiency is a common cause of anemia in otherwise healthy individuals and plays an important role in the development of anemia within the heart failure patient population. Iron-deficient heart failure patients experience worse symptoms and are less exercise tolerant than those without iron deficiency. These symptoms may occur even before clinical anemia is evident. This article reviews studies of the benefits of the use of intravenous iron to treat iron deficiency in anemic and nonanemic heart failure patients and an overview of the physiology and pathophysiology of iron metabolism in chronic heart failure.

Erythropoiesis Stimulation in Acute Ischemic Syndromes   313

Willem-Peter T. Ruifrok, Erik Lipšic, Rudolf A. de Boer, Wiek H. van Gilst, and Dirk J. van Veldhuisen

Erythropoietin (EPO) is a hematopoietic hormone with extensive nonhematopoietic properties. The discovery of an EPO receptor outside the hematopoietic system has fuelled research into the beneficial effects of EPO for various conditions, predominantly in cardiovascular disease. Experimental evidence has revealed the cytoprotective properties of EPO, and it seems that the EPO-EPO receptor system provides a powerful backbone against acute myocardial ischemia, gaining from the different properties of EPO. There is an ongoing discussion about possible discrepancy between preclinical and clinical effects of EPO on the cardiovascular system. Large, randomized, placebo-controlled clinical trials are underway to give a final verdict on EPO treatment for acute coronary syndromes.

Therapy with Erythropoiesis-Stimulating Agents and Renal and Nonrenal Outcomes   323

Anil K. Agarwal and Ajay K. Singh

The effect of erythropoiesis-stimulating agents (ESAs) on renal and cardiovascular outcomes in patients with chronic kidney disease (CKD) and heart failure (HF) is uncertain. Observational data indicate a strong relationship between the severity of anemia and poor outcome. On the other hand, randomized controlled trials on patients with CKD indicate that ESAs used in targeting a higher hemoglobin concentration result in increased risk. This article reviews the observational data as well as the recent information from randomized trials that point to increased risk in CKD and HF settings, and whether these disparate results can be explained by exposure to ESAs in this setting.

Epidemiology of Cardiorenal Syndrome   333

Robert J. Mentz and Eldrin F. Lewis

The interdependence of cardiac and renal dysfunction has emerged as a focus of intense interest in heart failure management due to the substantial associated morbidity and mortality. Captured in the clinical entity known as cardiorenal syndrome, recent definitions afford discussion of the acute and longitudinal evaluation and management of these patients. This article discusses potential pathophysiologic mechanisms of cardiorenal syndrome, epidemiology, inpatient and long-term care (including investigational therapies and mechanical fluid removal), and end-of-life and palliative care.

Anemia in Chronic Kidney Disease: New Advances   347

Tejas V. Patel and Ajay K. Singh

Anemia resulting from iron and erythropoietin deficiencies is a common complication of advanced chronic kidney disease (CKD). This article covers major advances in our understanding of anemia in patients with CKD, including newly discovered regulatory molecules, such as hepcidin, to innovative intravenous iron therapies. The use of erythropoiesis-stimulating agents (ESA) in the treatment of anemia has undergone seismic shift in the past 3 years as a result of adverse outcomes associated with targeting higher hemoglobin levels with these agents. Potential mechanisms for adverse outcomes, such as higher mortality, are discussed. Despite the disappointing experience with ESAs, there is a tremendous interest in other novel agents to treat anemia in CKD. Lastly, while awaiting updated guidelines, the authors outline their recommendations on how to best manage patients who are anemic and have CKD.

Outcomes Associated with Anemia in Patients with Heart Failure   359

Adam C. Salisbury and Mikhail Kosiborod

Over the past decade, a growing body of literature has led to a greater understanding of the relationship between anemia and the outcomes in patients with heart failure. This article reviews the current literature on the association between anemia and a broad range of clinical outcomes, including mortality, hospitalization, health status, and cost.

The Economic Burden of Anemia in Heart Failure   373

Richard K. Spence

Anemia is a complex issue in patients with heart failure (HF). In past years, clinicians accepted anemia as a given or an "accessory" diagnosis in HF patients. This attitude has changed since understanding of the causes and morbidity of anemia in HF has improved and with the introduction of targeted treatments. Increasing health care costs have stimulated vigorous debate about the cost-effectiveness of such treatments. It behooves clinicians to understand the effectiveness of specific treatments, risks and benefits, and costs. This review addresses the impact of anemia's prevalence, etiology, associated outcomes, and treatments on the economic burden of HF patients.

Future Directions in Management of Anemia in Heart Failure   385

Anil K. Agarwal and Stuart D. Katz

Anemia in patients with heart failure (HF) may be caused by several factors, including hemodilution, iron or erythropoietin deficiency, and chronic kidney disease.

Published pilot studies of erythropoiesis-stimulating agents (ESAs) and intravenous iron therapy in anemic heart failure patients demonstrate improvement in surrogate markers of functional capacity and quality of life, and reasonable safety profile during short-term use. However, the long-term safety of ESA in treatment of anemia in patients with HF remains a concern due to documented harmful side effects of ESA in anemic patients with advanced chronic kidney disease and cancer. Ongoing prospective clinical outcomes studies of ESA and intravenous iron therapies will provide important data that may pave the way for new avenues in the treatment of anemia in the future.

Index   **397**

Heart Failure Clinics

FORTHCOMING ISSUES

October 2010

Heart Failure in Children
Jeffrey A. Towbin, MD,
Guest Editor

January 2011

Depression and Heart Failure
Philip F. Binkley, MD, MPH,
and Stephen Gottlieb, MD,
Guest Editors

April 2011

Sudden Cardiac Death and Heart Failure
Raul Weiss, MD, and Emile Daoud, MD,
Guest Editors

RECENT ISSUES

April 2010

Genetics of Cardiomyopathy and Heart Failure
Calum A. MacRae, MD, PhD,
Guest Editor

January 2010

Pharmacogenetics in Heart Failure: How It Will Shape the Future
Dennis M. McNamara, MD, *Guest Editor*

October 2009

Biomarkers in Heart Failure
Eugene Braunwald, MD,
Guest Editor

ISSUES OF RELATED INTEREST

Cardiology Clinics May 2010 (Volume 28, Issue 2)
Controversies in Diseases of the Aorta
John A. Elefteriades, MD, *Guest Editor*
Available at: http://www.cardiology.theclinics.com/

Cardiology Clinics February 2010 (Volume 28, Issue 1)
Advanced Applied Interventional Cardiology
Samin K. Sharma, MD, FSCAI, FACC, and Annapoorna S. Kini, MD, MRCP, FACC,
Guest Editors
Available at: http://www.cardiology.theclinics.com/

VISIT THE CLINICS ONLINE!

Access your subscription at:
www.theclinics.com

Editorial
Staying in the Pink of Health for Patients with Cardiorenal Anemia Requires a Multidisciplinary Approach

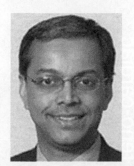 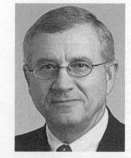

Ragavendra R. Baliga, MD, MBA   James B. Young, MD

Consulting Editors

Anemia in heart failure is not only debilitating but also associated with higher morbidity, mortality, and greater total health care costs[1] In an ever-aging population. It is common in patients who have heart failure, with a prevalence ranging from 4% to 55%.[2] Most studies indicate that the prevalence of anemia is higher in patients with heart failure who are more symptomatic or have comorbid conditions, such as kidney disease, diabetes mellitus, and advanced age, when compared with ambulatory and less-symptomatic patients.[3,4] The relative risk of death increases by a factor of 1.6 in anemic patients with heart failure who also have chronic kidney disease.

The pathophysiology of cardiorenal failure is multifactorial.[5] A recent consensus conference on cardiorenal syndromes[6] described 5 subtypes with distinct pathophysiologies (**Fig. 1**),[7] prevention, and management strategies (**Fig. 2**):

- Type 1, or acute cardiorenal syndrome, is acute worsening of heart function leading to kidney injury or dysfunction. Approximately 27% to 40% of the patients with acute decompensated heart failure seem to develop acute kidney injury. This type is associated with the poorest prognosis.
- Type 2, or chronic cardiorenal syndrome, includes patients with chronic abnormalities in heart function leading to kidney injury or

dysfunction. This has been reported in 63% of patients hospitalized with congestive heart failure. In this subset, serum creatinine may not entirely reflect underlying renal function.
- Type 3, or acute renocardiac syndrome, is acute worsening of kidney function, leading to heart injury or dysfunction. The effects on heart function are due to factors in addition to volume overload (eg, acute kidney injury, glomerulonephritis, and renal ischemia).
- Type 4, or chronic renocardiac syndrome, is a situation in which chronic kidney disease leads to heart injury, disease, or dysfunction (eg, chronic glomerulonephritis).
- Type 5, or secondary cardiorenal syndrome, includes systemic conditions leading to injury or dysfunction of heart and kidney (eg, diabetes mellitus, sepsis, systemic lupus erythematosus, or amyloidosis).

Patients may move from one subtype to another depending on the nature of primary insult. The recognition of these 5 distinct subtypes of cardiorenal failure should facilitate better understanding not only of these conditions but also of accompanying comorbidities, such as anemia.

The etiology and pathophysiology of anemia in heart failure is also multifactorial[8] and is due to a complex interaction[9] between cardiac function, renal dysfunction, neurohormonal and inflammatory

Heart Failure Clin 6 (2010) xi–xvi
doi:10.1016/j.hfc.2010.05.001
1551-7136/10/$ – see front matter © 2010 Elsevier Inc. All rights reserved.

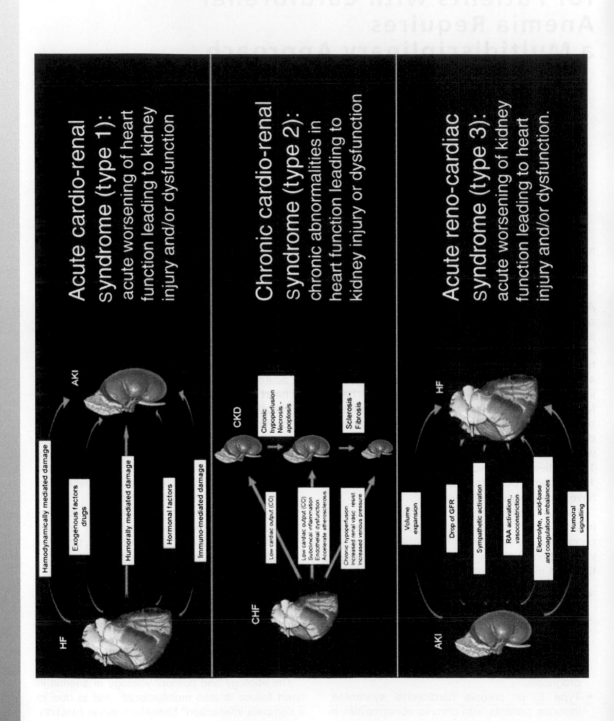

Acute cardio-renal syndrome (type 1): acute worsening of heart function leading to kidney injury and/or dysfunction

HF

AKI

Hamodynamically mediated damage

Exogenous factors
drugs

Humorally mediated damage

Hormonal factors

Immuno-mediated damage

Chronic cardio-renal syndrome (type 2): chronic abnormalities in heart function leading to kidney injury or dysfunction

CKD

CHF

Chronic
hypoperfusion
Necrosis -
apoptosis

Sclerosis -
Fibrosis

Low cardiac output (CO)

Low cardiac output (CO)
Subclinical inflammation
Endothelial dysfunction
Accelerate afterosclerosis.

Chronic hypoperfusion
Increased renal vasc. resist
Increased venous pressure

Acute reno-cardiac syndrome (type 3): acute worsening of kidney function leading to heart injury and/or dysfunction.

HF

AKI

Volume
expansion

Drop of GFR

Sympathetic activation

RAA activation.,
vasoconstriction

Electrolyte, acid-base
and coagulation imbalances

Humoral
signalling

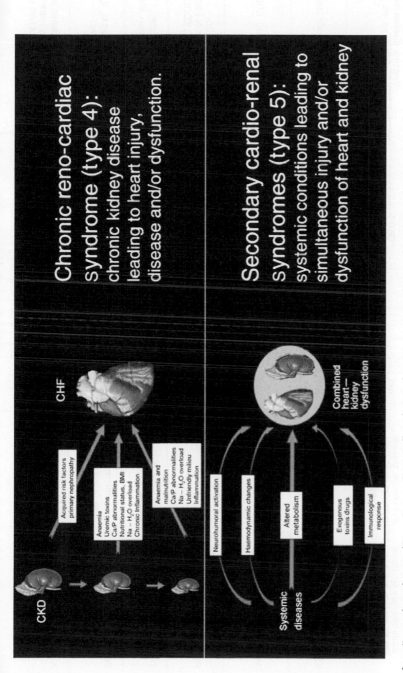

Fig. 1. Subtypes of cardiorenal syndrome. (*From* Ronco C, McCullough P, Anker SD, et al. Cardio-renal syndromes: report from the consensus conference of the acute dialysis quality initiative. Eur Heart J 2010;31(6):703–11; with permission.)

Syndromes	Acute cardio-renal (type 1)	Chronic cardio-renal (type 2)	Acute reno-cardiac (type 3)	Chronic reno-cardiac (type 4)	Secondary CRS (type 5)
Organ failure sequence					
Definition	Acute worsening of heart function (AHF–ACS) leading to kidney injury and/or dysfunction	Chronic abnormalities in heart function (CHF-CHD) leading to kidney injury or dysfunction	Acute worsening of kidney function (AKI) leading to heart injury and/or dysfunction	Chronic kidney disease (CKD) leading to heart injury, disease and/or dysfunction	Systemic conditions leading to simultaneous injury and/or dysfunction of heart and kidney
Primary events	Acute heart failure (AHF) or acute coronary syndrome (ACS) or cardiogenic shock	Chronic heart disease (LV remodelling and dysfunction, diastolic dysfunction, chronic abnormalities in cardiac function, cardiomyopathy)	AKI	CKD	Systemic disease (sepsis, amyloidosis, etc.)
Criteria for primary events	ESC, AHA/ACC	ESC, AHA/ACC	RIFLE–AKIN	KDOQI	Disease-specific criteria
Secondary events	AKI	CKD	AHF, ACS, arrhythmias, shock	CHD (LV remodelling and dysfunction, diastolic dysfunction, abnormalities in cardiac function), AHF, ACS	AHF, ACS, AKI, CHD, CKD
Criteria for secondary events	RIFLE–AKIN	KDOQI	ESC, AHA/ACC	ESC, AHA/ACC	ESC, AHA/ACC, RIFLE/AKIN ESC, AHA/ACC KDOQI
Cardiac biomarkers	Troponin, CK-MB, BNP, NT-proBNP, MPO, IMA	BNP, NT-proBNP, C-reactive protein	BNP, NT-proBNP	BNP, NT-proBNP, C-reactive protein	C-reactive protein, procalcitonin, BNP
Renal biomarkers	Serum cystatine C, creatinine, NGAL. Urinary KIM-1, IL-18, NGAL, NAG	Serum creatinine, cystatin C, urea, uric acid, C-reactive protein, decreased GFR	Serum creatinine, cystatin C, NGAL. Urinary KIM-1, IL-18, NGAL, NAG	Serum creatinine, cystatin C, urea, uric acid, decreased GFR	Creatinine, NGAL, IL-18, KIM-1, NAG
Prevention strategies	Acutely decompensated heart failure and acute coronary syndromes are	A common pathophysiology (neurohumoral, inflammatory, oxidative	Acute sodium and volume overload are part of the pathogenesis.	The chronic processes of cardiac and renal fibrosis, left ventricular hypertrophy,	Potential systemic factors negatively impact function of both organs

Syndromes	Acute cardio-renal (type 1)	Chronic cardio-renal (type 2)	Acute reno-cardiac (type 3)	Chronic reno-cardiac (type 4)	Secondary CRS (type 5)
	most common scenarios Inciting event may be acute coronary ischaemia, poorly controlled blood pressure, and noncompliance with medication and dietary sodium intake Randomized trials improving compliance with heart failure care management have reduced rates of hospitalization and mortality, and a reduction in the rates of acute cardio-renal syndrome (type 1) can be inferred	injury) could be at work to create organ dysfunction. Drugs that block the renin–angiotensin system reduce the progression of both heart failure and CKD It is unknown whether other classes of drugs can prevent chronic cardio-renal syndrome (type 2)	It is unknown whether sodium and volume overload is prevented with different forms of renal replacement therapy and if this will result in lower rates of cardiac decompensation	vascular stiffness, chronic Na and volume overload, and other factors (neurohumoral, inflammatory, oxidative injury) could be at work to create organ dysfunction A reduction in the decline of renal function and albuminuria has been associated with a reduction in cardiovascular events The role of chronic uraemia, anaemia, and changes in CKD-mineral and bone disorder on the cardiovascular system is known in chronic reno-cardiac syndrome	acutely. It is uncertain if reduction/elimination of the key factors (immune, inflammatory, oxidative stress, thrombosis) will prevent both cardiac and renal decline.
Management strategies	Specific—depends on precipitating factors General supportive—oxygenate, relieve pain & pulmonary congestion, treat arrhythmias appropriately, differentiate left from right heart failure, treat low cardiac output or congestion according to ESC guidelines[a], avoid nephrotoxins, closely monitor kidney function.	Treat CHF according to ESC guidelines[a], exclude precipitating pre-renal AKI factors (hypovolaemia and/or hypotension), adjust therapy accordingly and avoid nephrotoxins, while monitoring renal function and electrolytes. Extracorporeal ultrafiltration	Follow ESC guidelines for acute CHF[a] specific management may depend on underlying aetiology, may need to exclude renovascular disease and consider early renal support, if diuretic resistant	Follow KDOQI guidelines for CKD management, exclude precipitating causes (cardiac tamponade). Treat heart failure according to ESC guidelines[a], consider early renal replacement support	Specific—according to etiology. General—see CRS management as advised by ESC guidelines[a] 2008

Fig. 2. Cardiorenal syndromes: classification, definitions, and work group statements. ACC, American College of Cardiology; ACS, acute coronary syndrome; ADHF, acute de-compensated heart failure; ADQI, Acute Dialysis Quality Initiative; AHA, American Heart Association; AHF, acute heart failure; AKI, acute kidney injury; AKIN, Acute Kidney Injury Network; CHF, chronic heart failure; CKD, chronic kidney disease; KDOQI, Kidney Disease Outcome Quality Initiative; KIM-1, kidney injury molecule-1; MPO, myeloperoxidase; NAG, N-acetyl-b-(D)glucosaminidase; NGAL, neutrophil gelatinase-associated lipocalin; NKF, National Kidney Foundation; RIFLE, risk, injury, failure, loss of kidney function, and end-stage kidney disease; WRF, worsening renal function. [a] As advised by European Society of Cardiology guidelines 2008. (From Ronco C, McCullough P, Anker SD, et al. Cardio-renal syndromes: report from the consensus conference of the acute dialysis quality initiative. Eur Heart J 2010;31(6):703–11; with permission.)

responses, hemodilution, iron deficiency, impaired ability to use available iron stores,[10] bone marrow suppression due to cytokines (eg, tumor necrosis factor α [TNF-α], interleukin [IL]-1, IL-6, and C-reactive protein), blunted bone marrow responsiveness to erythropoietin, impaired iron mobilization, and effects of medications. Aspirin and angiotensin-converting enzyme inhibitors[11] contribute to the anemia potentially through the actions of hematopoesis inhibitor, N-acetyl-seryl-aspartyl-lysyl-proline.[12] IL-6 stimulates the production of hepcidin in the hepatic cells, which blocks absorption of iron in duodenum and down-regulates ferroprotein expression, which in turn prevents release of iron from total body stores.[13] In contrast, TNF-α and IL-6 inhibit erythropoietin production in the kidney by activating the GATA-binding protein, GATA2, and nuclear factor κB and also inhibits proliferation of bone marrow erythroid progenitor cells.[3,4,13] Some have used erythropoietin receptor–stimulating agents or intravenous iron to correct the anemia of heart failure, but concern has arisen about the true effectiveness of this approach and morbidity associated with the therapy. The Reduction of Events with Darbopoeitin Alfa in Heart Failure is a large-scale, phase III, placebo-controlled, randomized, morbidity and mortality clinical trial designed to clarify these issues and will likely be finished recruiting in 18 months.[14]

To unravel these complex interactions in cardiorenal anemia, Anil Agarwal, MD, Stuart Katz, MD, and Ajay Singh, MD, have assembled a multidisciplinary team of experts in this field. In our opinion, their multidisciplinary approach is essential to ensure that patients with cardiorenal anemia stay in the pink of health.

Ragavendra R. Baliga, MD, MBA
Division of Cardiovascular Medicine
The Ohio State University
Columbus, OH, USA

James B. Young, MD
Division of Medicine and Lerner
College of Medicine, Cleveland Clinic
Cleveland, OH, USA

E-mail addresses:
Ragavendra.Baliga@osumc.edu (R.R. Baliga)
YOUNGJ@ccf.org (J.B. Young)

REFERENCES

1. Allen LA, Anstrom KJ, Horton JR, et al. Relationship between anemia and health care costs in heart failure. J Card Fail 2009;15(10):843–9.
2. Tanner H, Moschovitis G, Kuster GM, et al. The prevalence of anemia in chronic heart failure. Int J Cardiol 2002;86(1):115–21.
3. Anand IS. Anemia and chronic heart failure implications and treatment options. J Am Coll Cardiol 2008; 52(7):501–11.
4. Dec GW. Anemia and iron deficiency–new therapeutic targets in heart failure? N Engl J Med 2009; 361(25):2475–7.
5. Baliga RR, Young JB. "Stiff central arteries" syndrome: does a weak heart really stiff the kidney? Heart Fail Clin 2008;4(4):ix–xii.
6. Ronco C, McCullough P, Anker SD, et al. Cardiorenal syndromes: report from the consensus conference of the acute dialysis quality initiative. Eur Heart J 2010;31(6):703–11.
7. Ronco C, Haapio M, House AA, et al. Cardiorenal syndrome. J Am Coll Cardiol 2008;52(19):1527–39.
8. Nanas JN, Matsouka C, Karageorgopoulos D, et al. Etiology of anemia in patients with advanced heart failure. J Am Coll Cardiol 2006;48(12):2485–9.
9. Felker GM. Too much, too little, or just right?: untangling endogenous erythropoietin in heart failure. Circulation 2010; 121(2):191–3.
10. Opasich C, Cazzola M, Scelsi L, et al. Blunted erythropoietin production and defective iron supply for erythropoiesis as major causes of anaemia in patients with chronic heart failure. Eur Heart J 2005;26(21): 2232–7.
11. Ishani A, Weinhandl E, Zhao Z, et al. Angiotensin-converting enzyme inhibitor as a risk factor for the development of anemia, and the impact of incident anemia on mortality in patients with left ventricular dysfunction. J Am Coll Cardiol 2005; 45(3):391–9.
12. van der Meer P, Lipsic E, Westenbrink BD, et al. Levels of hematopoiesis inhibitor N-acetyl-seryl-aspartyl-lysyl-proline partially explain the occurrence of anemia in heart failure. Circulation 2005;112(12):1743–7.
13. Weiss G, Goodnough LT. Anemia of chronic disease. N Engl J Med 2005;352(10):1011–23.
14. McMurray JJV, Anand IS, Diaz R, et al. Design of the reduction of events with darbepoetin alfa in heart failure (RED-HF): a phase III, anaemia correction, morbidity-morality trial. Eur J Heart Fail 2009;11: 795–801.

Preface

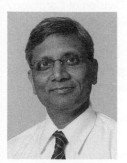
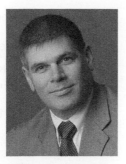
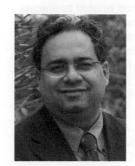

Anil K. Agarwal, MD   Stuart D. Katz, MD   Ajay K. Singh, MB, FRCP(UK)

Guest Editors

Anemia is common in patients with heart failure and defines a group of patients at very high risk for death and cardiovascular complications, particularly when diabetes mellitus, chronic kidney disease, or both are also present. The etiology of anemia in heart failure is complex and multifactorial. The mediators of risk are still being elucidated.

The introduction in 1989 of epoetin alfa as the first of now several erythropoiesis-stimulating agents (ESAs) has transformed the treatment of anemia. ESA therapy is currently used in treating anemia in patients with chronic kidney disease, cancer- and chemotherapy-induced anemia, heart failure, critical illness, or HIV/AIDS. Newer ESAs are being developed. Promising indications for ESA therapy include prevention of myocardial ischemia, cerebral ischemia, and acute kidney injury; trials are ongoing. Treatment of iron deficiency has also become an important component of managing anemia in heart failure. Several new intravenous iron preparations are emerging.

Many questions, however, remain unanswered. The mechanism of anemia in heart failure continues to be debated. The optimal diagnostic approach and treatment strategy for anemia in heart failure have not been determined. The divergent results derived from observational treatment studies and prospective randomized controlled trials have raised questions about the current guideline recommendations for treatment of anemia in patients with chronic kidney disease. Controversy abounds about whether or not treatment of anemia in heart failure with ESAs or iron is beneficial. A large prospective randomized trial in anemic heart failure patients, Reduction of Events with Darbepoetin alfa in Heart Failure (RED-HF), is ongoing. Concern remains that the risk of ESAs observed in treating anemia in kidney disease and cancer could apply to heart failure patients. In addition, concerns have been raised about the potential risk of increased oxidative stress conferred by intravenous iron preparations.

In this issue of *Heart Failure Clinics*, our goal is to bring together experts in anemia, kidney disease, and heart failure to address advanced and hot button issues in anemia and heart failure. The epidemiology of anemia in heart failure and the prevalence of cardiorenal syndrome are discussed to highlight the impact of kidney involvement on progression of anemia and worsening of the outcomes of heart failure. The current state of understanding of the pathophysiologic mechanisms of anemia, the role of treatment with ESA and iron, and the potential risks, benefits, and costs associated with treatment of anemia in heart failure are also elaborated. Finally, we speculate on future directions in the management of anemia in heart failure and novel application of ESA therapies in other cardiovascular disease states.

Heart Failure Clin 6 (2010) xvii–xviii
doi:10.1016/j.hfc.2010.04.001
1551-7136/10/$ – see front matter © 2010 Elsevier Inc. All rights reserved.

The overall aim of this issue is to provide mechanistic and clinical perspectives related to anemia of heart failure based on available evidence. We will have succeeded if readers and colleagues are left with the impression that this is a dynamic area with much opportunity for further investigation and inquiry.

Anil K. Agarwal, MD
Division of Nephrology
The Ohio State University
395 West 12th Avenue, Ground Floor
Columbus, OH 43210, USA

Stuart D. Katz, MD
Division of Cardiology
NYU Langone Medical Center, Skirball 9R
550 First Avenue
New York, NY 10016, USA

Ajay K. Singh, MB, FRCP(UK)
Brigham and Women's Hospital
75 Francis Street
Boston, MA 02115, USA

E-mail addresses:
anil.agarwal@osumc.edu (A.K. Agarwal)
stuart.katz@nyumc.org (S.D. Katz)
asingh@rics.bwh.harvard.edu (A.K. Singh)

Epidemiology of Anemia in Heart Failure

W.H. Wilson Tang, MD[a],*,
P.S. Daniel Yeo, MBBS, MRCP(UK)[b]

KEYWORDS

• Anemia • Heart failure • Epidemiology

Over the past decade, there has been increasing recognition of the importance of anemia in the pathophysiology, treatment, and prognosis of heart failure. Anemia was once considered a downstream, comorbid complication largely related to progressive renal insufficiency or a rare but reversible cause of high-output heart failure. There is now an emerging appreciation that targeting anemia may serve as a potential treatment strategy for patients with chronic heart failure. This article focuses on the contemporary epidemiology of anemia based on observations from different settings of heart failure.

DEFINITION

Determining how common anemia is in patients with heart failure depends on how anemia is defined. It also varies according to the setting and population in which anemia is being considered. The precise cutoffs to define anemia in heart failure are largely philosophic, and there is no consensus as to the definition of anemia specific to patients with heart failure. Some investigators follow the historical definition of anemia that was put forward by the World Health Organization (WHO) in the discussion of nutritional anemia over 4 decades ago, namely hemoglobin (Hb) concentration less than 13 g/dL for men or less than 12 g/dL for women.[1] However, such a definition has not been subjected to rigorous clinical

validation of its significance, particularly in the setting of heart failure, and its appropriateness and clinical applicability continues to be debated.[2] In their latest guidelines, the National Kidney Foundation modified their original gender-independent cutoff of 12 g/dL to define the presence of anemia with Hb less than 13.5 g/dL for men or less than 12 g/dL for women, largely raising the cutoff to increase the awareness of the diagnosis and management of anemia in the setting of renal insufficiency because more patients are considered anemic with this broader definition,[3] Other investigators prefer to use a more conservative definition (eg, <12 g/dL for men and <11 g/dL for women) to ensure that a higher confidence in capturing the affected patient population can be achieved.[4,5] Patients with heart failure can have anemia as a true comorbid condition unrelated to the heart failure syndrome (eg, in the setting of gastrointestinal bleeding) rather than as a specific clinical entity associated with the pathophysiology of heart failure.

The contemporary understanding of anemia in heart failure is highly dependent on the specific setting in which hematologic data were made available. As reports regarding anemia, specifically in chronic heart failure populations, were derived from post hoc analyses from multicenter drug trials that collected information about a single value of hematocrit (Hct) as adjunct data (eg, to determine safety to obtain blood

Financial disclosure: No relationships to disclose.
[a] Section of Heart Failure and Cardiac Transplantation Medicine, Heart and Vascular Institute, Cleveland Clinic, 9500 Euclid Avenue, Desk J3-4, Cleveland, OH 44195, USA
[b] Department of Cardiovascular Medicine, Tan Tock Seng Hospital, 11 Jalan Tan Tock Seng, Singapore 308433, Republic of Singapore
* Corresponding author. Section of Heart Failure and Cardiac Transplantation Medicine, Heart and Vascular Institute, Cleveland Clinic, 9500 Euclid Avenue, Desk J3-4, Cleveland, OH 44195.
E-mail address: tangw@ccf.org

Heart Failure Clin 6 (2010) 271–278
doi:10.1016/j.hfc.2010.03.007
1551-7136/10/$ – see front matter © 2010 Elsevier Inc. All rights reserved.

draws or whether the investigational drug was interfering with hematologic processes), a parallel definition based on Hct has evolved. Although overall Hb and Hct levels correlate well in direct comparisons, criteria defined by Hct may identify more patients with a diagnosis of anemia.[6] A range of cutoff values (between 35% and 39%) have been reported in the literature.[7–9]

It is equally important to recognize that anemia is often overlooked by health care providers, and therefore defining anemia by International Classification of Diseases (ICD)-9 codes may underestimate the true prevalence when directly compared with actual Hb or Hct measurements. In a large tertiary care practice, the documentation of anemia as a clinical diagnosis as well as a diagnostic workup in the electronic health record was uncommon.[5] Internal medicine clinics, being more in tune to work up various medical problems, have demonstrated a greater likelihood of listing anemia as a clinical diagnosis than cardiology clinics. This failure to clinically diagnose anemia may be because cardiology clinics health care providers often focus on immediate needs to monitor cardiorenal status and may not routinely perform a complete blood count.

PREVALENCE

Anemia is prevalent in patients with heart failure regardless of the clinical setting, although the exact rates vary widely. **Table 1** provides an overview of the major reports on the prevalence of anemia over the past decade. A recent meta-analysis analyzed a total of 153,180 patients with heart failure reported in 34 published studies from 2001 to 2007 and estimated the prevalence of anemia to be 37.2%.[27] This finding is consistent with the findings from the latest prospective STAMINA-HFP (Study of Anemia in a Heart Failure Population) Registry, which identified a prevalence of 34% in a cohort of 1076 unselected outpatients with chronic heart failure (based on WHO criteria).[10] Hence, the prevalence of anemia in a heart failure population likely ranges from one-fifth to one-third of patients.

Beyond variations in definitions, it is not surprising that different practice settings have vastly different rates, with those patients in the acute decompensated states likely experiencing more dilutional anemia. In a Scottish admission registry, with testing performed within 24 hours of admission, 51% of men and 45% of women were anemic as defined

Table 1
Prevalence of anemia in heart failure from selected large major studies

Study	Definition	No. of Patients	Prevalence
Val-HeFT[15]	Hb <11 g/dL (F), <12 g/dL (M)	5010	10%
COMET[14]	Hb <12 g/dL (F), <13 g/dL (M)	3029	16%
IN-CHF[4]	Hb <11 g/dL (F), <12 g/dL (M)	2411	16%
Ezekowitz et al[11]	ICD-9 codes	12065	17%
Tang et al[5]	Hb <11 g/dL (F), <12 g/dL (M)	6055	17%
ELITE-II[36]	Hb ≤12.4 g/dL	3044	17%
RENAISSANCE[23]	Hb ≤12 g/dL	912	20%
PRAISE[9]	Hct <37.6%	1130	20%
EuroHeart Failure Survey[37]	Hb <11 g/dL	9971	21%
CHARM[21]	Hb <12 g/dL (F), <13 g/dL (M)	2653	26%
Herzog et al[38]	ICD-9 code	152584	28%
Horwich et al[28]	Hb <12 g/dL (F), <13 g/dL (M)	1061	30%
STAMINA-HFP[10]	Hb <12 g/dL (F), <13 g/dL (M)	982	33%
Kosiborod et al[30]	Hct ≤37%	2281	48%
OPTIME-CHF[39]	Hb <12 g/dL (F), <13 g/dL (M)	906	49%

Abbreviations: CHARM, Candesartan in Heart Failure: Assessment of Reduction in Mortality and Morbidity; COMET, Carvedilol or Metoprolol European Trial; ELITE-II, Evaluation of Losartan In The Elderly—II; F, female; IN-CHF, Italian Network on Congestive Heart Failure; M, male; OPTIME-CHF, Outcomes of a Prospective Trial of Intravenous Milrinone for Exacerbations of Chronic Heart Failure; PRAISE, Prospective Randomized Amlodipine Survival Evaluation; RENAISSANCE, Randomized Etanercept North America Strategy to Study Antagonism of Cytokines; STAMINA-HFP, Study of Anemia in a Heart Failure Population; Val-HeFT, Valsartan in Heart Failure Trial.

by Hb less than 12 g/dL.[6] By Hct criteria, 57% of men and 47% of women were anemic. Among patients who were anemic by Hb criteria, 81% had normal, 10% had low, and 9% had increased mean red blood cell volume. In contrast, those enrolled in clinical trials may have less severe forms as a result of exclusion criteria for severe anemia or advanced renal insufficiency. Overall, the prevalence of anemia varies widely, ranging from 14% to 56% in outpatient registries, from 14% to 61% in hospitalized patients, and from 4% to 49% in clinical trial databases. The general consensus is that large observational databases have provided the most consistent estimates of anemia in a real-world setting, despite various definitions for anemia. An unselected population-based cohort of 12,065 patients with new-onset heart failure identified from Canadian hospital discharges had an anemia prevalence of 17%, among whom 58% were classified as having anemia of chronic disease based on ICD-9 coding.[11] This prevalence rate was consistent with a 17% prevalence rate observed in a large and diverse ambulatory patient population with chronic heart failure.[5] By contrast, a large, retrospective, observational, longitudinal cohort study of 59,772 patients in the Kaiser Permanente Health System with at least 1 admission with heart failure as one of the diagnoses showed an anemia prevalence as high as 42.6%.[12] Whether this was because of a selected group of patients who had advanced diseases (who warranted hospitalization) was not elaborated.

Even though anemia can be prevalent, the severity of anemia is usually mild and can be easily overlooked. In STAMINA-HFP, significant anemia was not commonly observed, as illustrated by only about 12% of total population having Hb less than 11 g/dL (**Fig. 1**). The use of a single cutoff value for determining the presence of anemia is also problematic because small changes around the cutoff value(s) may greatly alter the calculations of prevalence rates.

INCIDENCE

Few registry studies have reported on the incidence of anemia in patients with heart failure because few studies included serial assessment of Hb or Hct levels. In contrast, large clinical trials lend themselves well to understanding the incidence of anemia because of their prospective design and close follow-up. That being said, determining the incidence of anemia in heart failure

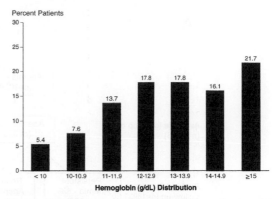

Fig. 1. Distribution of hemoglobin in patients with chronic heart failure: STAMINA-HFP. (*Adapted from* Adams KF Jr, Patterson JH, Oren RM, et al. Prospective assessment of the occurrence of anemia in patients with heart failure: results from the Study of Anemia in a Heart Failure Population (STAMINA-HFP) Registry. Am Heart J 2009;157:926; with permission.)

clinical trial participants can be biased because of the exclusion of subjects with significant anemia or preexisting renal insufficiency. The Studies of Left Ventricular Dysfunction (SOLVD) Trial found a 9.6% 1-year incidence of new-onset anemia.[13] More recent large trials such as Carvedilol or Metoprolol European Trial and the Valsartan in Heart Failure Trial (Val-HeFT) observed higher 1-year incidence rates of 14.2%[14] and 16.9%,[15] respectively. The incidence of real-world new-onset anemia may even be higher, with up to 20% over a 6-month follow-up period in 1070 ambulatory patients with chronic heart failure.[5] Because the volume status of the patients at baseline was not well characterized, the true incidence can be influenced by dilutional anemia as a result of hypervolemia in congested patients, which may resolve after stabilization and treatment.[8] Furthermore, for those with anemia at baseline (n = 323), 43% demonstrated resolution of anemia (so-called transient anemia, **Fig. 2** upper panel). With fluctuating volume status, the true incidence may be difficult to ascertain in patients with heart failure. Nevertheless, patients who have less-impaired cardiac function (left ventricular ejection fraction [LVEF] >30%, B-type natriuretic peptide ≤325 pg/mL) or renal function (estimated glomerular filtration rate [GFR] ≥60 mL/min/1.73 m^2), as well as those without diabetes mellitus, were more likely to have their anemia resolved over time.

CAUSES AND CONFOUNDERS OF ANEMIA

There are many potential underlying causes of anemia in the setting of heart failure. The main causes of anemia in heart failure include nutritional

A

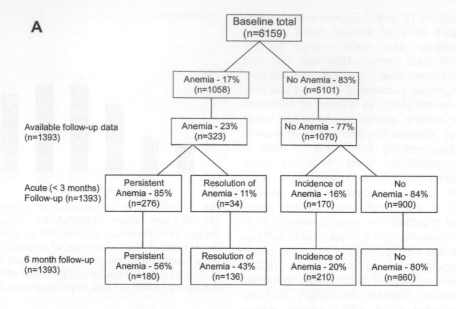

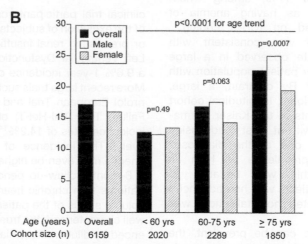

Fig. 2. Epidemiology of anemia in ambulatory patients with chronic heart failure. (*Adapted from* Tang WH, Tong W, Jain A, et al. Evaluation and long-term prognosis of new-onset, transient, and persistent anemia in ambulatory patients with chronic heart failure. J Am Coll Cardiol 2008;51:569; with permission.)

deficiencies (eg, malabsorption, impaired metabolism), acute blood loss (eg, gastrointestinal bleeding, although not a common occurrence[6]), intrinsic renal disease leading to insufficient erythropoietin production or response, or hemodilution from volume expansion. Most patients present with normocytic anemia,[5] with similar mean corpuscular volume across the spectrum of Hb levels.[10] These findings suggest that there is a relatively low prevalence of significant iron deficiency, even though the presence of functional or subclinical iron deficiency cannot be excluded. This low prevalence is particularly relevant in light of the recent demonstration of potential benefits of iron infusions in improving functional capacity in

patients with heart failure,[16] suggesting that relative iron deficiency may be present.

Heart Failure Disease Severity

The presence of anemia is tightly linked to clinical disease severity of heart failure. The presence of more advanced signs and symptoms of heart failure (noted as higher New York Heart Association Functional Class) was associated with greater prevalence of anemia.[5,15] The reasons for this prevalence can be multifactorial. Meanwhile, post hoc analysis of the data from clinical trials have provided a host of other factors which were all predictors of incident anemia, including more advanced age, higher dose of diuretics or the use of spironolactone and digoxin, elevated serum creatinine and potassium, as well as lower serum sodium and body mass index, which are all suggestive of worsening heart failure severity. This concept is supported by the fact that patients with higher plasma levels of natriuretic peptide demonstrated higher likelihood of presenting with anemia than those with lower levels of plasma natriuretic peptide.[5,15] Anemia has also been directly attributable to the chronic inflammatory disease state of heart failure itself, as a potential classification of "anemia of chronic disease."[17,18]

Demographic Data

Advancing age is an important contributor to the development of anemia. In an apparently healthy elderly population, the prevalence of anemia is around 10%, and can increase up to 20% in those older than 85 years.[19] As in non–heart failure settings, older patients with heart failure tend to have higher likelihood of developing future anemia (see **Fig. 2**, lower panel).

Although gender plays an important role in the overall prevalence of anemia in the general population, the prevalence and clinical consequences appeared to be similar in several reports in heart failure cohorts.[5,15] As age increases, the prevalence of anemia in men may even surpass than that in women, which balances out the higher prevalence of anemia in middle-aged women over middle-aged men (see **Fig. 2**, lower panel).[5] Meanwhile, Caucasian patients tend to have lower rates of anemia than non-Caucasian patients as observed in Val-HeFT,[15] but this may be because of potential selection bias from study populations and underlying comorbidities as major confounders.

The contribution of various other demographic factors to the development of anemia have been confirmed in STAMINA-HFP, in which 40% of ambulatory patients with heart failure who were older than 70 years demonstrated the presence of anemia.[10] In multivariable analysis, especially after adjusting for renal function, diastolic blood pressure, and presence of edema, age and gender were no longer independent predictors for the presence of anemia. However, African American ethnicity remained a predictor of anemia.

Preserved Versus Impaired Ejection Fraction

Several observational series have stratified patients according to their reported LVEF and have found similar prevalence in preserved and impaired LVEF.[6,15,20] Analysis of the Candesartan Heart Failure Assessment of Reduction in Mortality and Morbidity (CHARM) Program data also found that the prevalence of anemia was similar between those with preserved LVEF and reduced LVEF (27% and 25%, respectively) even though a weak inverse relation of Hb with LVEF was observed.[21] This observation is likely confounded with advancing age (favoring the development of anemia in those with preserved LVEF) as well as underlying organ dysfunction (favoring the development of anemia in those with impaired LVEF), although in Val-HeFT (restricted to impaired LVEF) the relationship between Hb and LVEF was less apparent.[15]

Meanwhile, the prevalence of diastolic dysfunction was directly proportional to the presence and severity of anemia (defined as Hb <13 g/dL, with severe anemia defined as Hb <11 g/dL). In a stable patient cohort undergoing cardiac catheterization, only 8% of nonanemics had diastolic dysfunction, whereas 13% of patients with mild to moderate anemia and 24% of patients with severe anemia had diastolic dysfunction.[22] Furthermore, Hb level correlated inversely with the presence of diastolic dysfunction ($P = .004$), with each 1 g/dL decrease in Hb giving a 40% higher odds ratio of diastolic dysfunction.[22] This study would have classified fewer patients as having diastolic dysfunction because patients with LVEF of less than 50% were excluded.

Diabetes Mellitus

Consistent across different observational cohorts, patients with a history of diabetes mellitus demonstrated greater prevalence of anemia than their nondiabetic counterparts.[5,10] Furthermore, patients with anemia had a higher prevalence of diabetes mellitus than nonanemic patients (Val-HeFT: 34% vs 23%, respectively, $P<.001$).[23]

Renal Insufficiency

Intrinsic renal disease leading to reduced erythropoietin production has been one of the predominant contributors to the development of anemia in patients with heart failure and concomitant renal insufficiency. The presence of impaired renal function (GFR <60 mL/min/1.73 m^2) was associated with a 3-fold higher likelihood of developing anemia.[5,6] In an analysis of the CHARM Program with a 26% prevalence of anemic patients, more than half had Stage III to IV chronic kidney disease compared with less than a third of nonanemic patients.[21] In particular, the degree of anemia was directly proportional to the degree of renal dysfunction, with every 10-point decrease of GFR below 60 mL/min/1.73 m^2 being associated with a decrease of Hb by 0.290 g/dL.

Hemodilution

Destabilized heart failure poses a unique environment to produce a so-called dilutional anemia caused by hypervolemia. A single-center report described a 46% prevalence of dilutional anemia in 37 patients referred for heart transplant workup based on careful blood volume analysis.[8] This finding may also explain why in a large cohort of anemic ambulatory patients with heart failure, a substantial proportion demonstrated resolution of their anemic status without specific intervention besides standard heart failure medications largely to achieve euvolemia.[5]

Chronic Inflammation

Although anemia in heart failure has often been attributed to some form of anemia of chronic disease, few studies have carefully analyzed the interplay between Hb or Hct and other inflammatory biomarkers. This interplay may explain why the presence of anemia has been associated with higher levels of high-sensitivity C-reactive protein.[15,24] It appears that inflammatory response as a contributor to the development of anemia may be more prominent in patients with ischemic heart failure.[25]

MORBIDITY AND MORTALITY

As expected, patients with anemia are more likely to be more symptomatic.[15] The most comprehensive evaluation regarding the impact of anemia on cardiovascular morbidity in patients with heart failure used quality-of-life questionnaires with serial assessment in the STAMINA-HFP Registry.[26] In particular, adjusted changes in Kansas City Cardiomyopathy Questionnaire clinical scores were significantly associated with change in Hb from baseline to 6 months (**Fig. 3**,

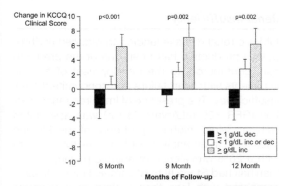

Fig. 3. Relation of changes in hemoglobin levels with health status assessment. (*Adapted from* Adams KF Jr, Pina IL, Ghali JK, et al. Prospective evaluation of the association between hemoglobin concentration and quality of life in patients with heart failure. Am Heart J 2009;158:965; with permission.)

lower panel). These findings concur with prior reports in Val-HeFT regarding higher Minnesota Living with Heart Failure Questionnaire scores with more advanced heart failure symptoms.[15] However, these observations do not provide insights into cause-effect relationships. The Val-HeFT Study found that patients who had the largest increase in Hb over 1 year were associated with slightly less improvement in left ventricular internal diastolic diameter and LVEF than others who had smaller increases or decreases in Hb.[23]

Consistent across the published literature, the presence of anemia is associated with poorer prognosis in patients with heart failure.[23,27,28] The SOLVD Study showed that mortality increased by 3% for every 1% decrease in Hct (approximate 10% increase in mortality for every Hb decrease of 1 g/dL).[7] Meanwhile, in a large retrospective evaluation of elderly patients with heart failure, the presence of anemia remained an independent predictor of heart failure readmissions (despite not for mortality) after adjusting for multiple comorbidities and clinical factors.[29] Data from the Val-HeFT trial on 5002 patients confirmed that the presence of anemia as well as new-onset anemia within a 12-month follow-up were independent predictors of long-term mortality.[15] Several other large studies in chronic heart failure population also showed an increase in mortality ranging from 8% to 16% for every Hb decrease of 1 g/dL.[12,15,23,28] Patients with the largest decrease in Hb levels had the worst rates for heart failure readmissions, mortality, and morbidity.[14] These associations are strong and may point to a causal relationship, but this observation is still an area of controversy because some studies did not find anemia to be an independent predictor for adverse outcomes.[18,30] (See the article by Salisbury and Kosiborod elsewhere in this issue for further exploration of this topic.)

One of the biggest limitations of database or post hoc analyses is reliance on a single time-point Hb or Hct measurement to be associated with long-term clinical outcomes. This approach assumes that the Hb and Hct measured are relatively stable. In reality, measurements of Hb or Hct can be quite dynamic, and several studies have documented the "transient" nature of a diagnosis of anemia in some patients, often associated with a more favorable prognosis.[5,15,31]

IMPACT ON DRUG THERAPY

In general, drug therapy that improves long-term outcomes has been associated with resolution of anemia or increase in Hb levels over time.[32] One big exception is angiotensin-converting enzyme inhibitors, which are known to cause approximately 0.5 g/dL reduction in Hb levels because of their ability to suppress erythropoietin synthesis.[33] This observation was illustrated in the SOLVD Study, in which enalapril increased the odds of incident anemia (Hct ≤39% in men or Hct ≤36% in women) at 1 year by 56% in adjusted models. Furthermore, those with prevalent or incident anemia had poorer prognosis, but the use of enalapril still demonstrated a survival benefit.[13] Similar findings were noted for angiotensin receptor blockers such as valsartan[15] or losartan[34] within a few months of therapy, though perhaps less apparent.[35] These findings illustrate that not all anemias translate to harm, and careful understanding of the underlying causes of anemia may provide better insights into their clinical significance.

SUMMARY

Anemia occurs frequently in a substantial proportion of patients with heart failure, often in mild, normocytic form. The condition's associations with comorbidities such as diabetes mellitus and renal sufficiency are clues to its potential underlying shared pathophysiology. Understanding the epidemiologic data can allow health care providers and researchers to appreciate the scope and consequences of the problem of anemia in the heart failure population and the need to develop strategies to address issues related to patient selection and treatment modalities.

REFERENCES

1. Blanc B, Finch CA, Hallberg L, et al. Nutritional anemias. Report of a WHO Scientific Group. World Health Organ Tech Rep Ser 1968;405:1.
2. Beutler E, Waalen J. The definition of anemia: what is the lower limit of normal of the blood hemoglobin concentration? Blood 2006;107:1747.
3. National Kidney Foundation. KDOQI Clinical Practice Guidelines and Clinical Practice Recommendations for Anemia in Chronic Kidney Disease. Am J Kidney Dis 2006;47:S1.
4. Maggioni AP, Opasich C, Anand I, et al. Anemia in patients with heart failure: prevalence and prognostic role in a controlled trial and in clinical practice. J Card Fail 2005;11:91.
5. Tang WH, Tong W, Jain A, et al. Evaluation and long-term prognosis of new-onset, transient, and persistent anemia in ambulatory patients with chronic heart failure. J Am Coll Cardiol 2008;51:569.
6. Berry C, Norrie J, Hogg K, et al. The prevalence, nature, and importance of hematologic abnormalities in heart failure. Am Heart J 2006;151:1313.
7. Al-Ahmad A, Rand WM, Manjunath G, et al. Reduced kidney function and anemia as risk factors for mortality in patients with left ventricular dysfunction. J Am Coll Cardiol 2001;38:955.
8. Androne AS, Katz SD, Lund L, et al. Hemodilution is common in patients with advanced heart failure. Circulation 2003;107:226.
9. Mozaffarian D, Nye R, Levy WC. Anemia predicts mortality in severe heart failure: the prospective randomized amlodipine survival evaluation (PRAISE). J Am Coll Cardiol 1933;41:2003.
10. Adams KF Jr, Patterson JH, Oren RM, et al. Prospective assessment of the occurrence of anemia in patients with heart failure: results from the Study of Anemia in a Heart Failure Population (STAMINA-HFP) Registry. Am Heart J 2009;157:926.
11. Ezekowitz JA, McAlister FA, Armstrong PW. Anemia is common in heart failure and is associated with poor outcomes: insights from a cohort of 12 065 patients with new-onset heart failure. Circulation 2003;107:223.
12. Go AS, Yang J, Ackerson LM, et al. Hemoglobin level, chronic kidney disease, and the risks of death and hospitalization in adults with chronic heart failure: the Anemia in Chronic Heart Failure: Outcomes and Resource Utilization (ANCHOR) Study. Circulation 2006;113:2713.
13. Ishani A, Weinhandl E, Zhao Z, et al. Angiotensin-converting enzyme inhibitor as a risk factor for the development of anemia, and the impact of incident anemia on mortality in patients with left ventricular dysfunction. J Am Coll Cardiol 2005;45:391.
14. Komajda M, Anker SD, Charlesworth A, et al. The impact of new onset anemia on morbidity and mortality in chronic heart failure: results from COMET. Eur Heart J 2006;27:1440.
15. Anand IS, Kuskowski MA, Rector TS, et al. Anemia and change in hemoglobin over time related to mortality and morbidity in patients with chronic heart failure: results from Val-HeFT. Circulation 2005;112:1121.
16. Anker SD, Comin Colet J, Filippatos G, et al. Ferric carboxymaltose in patients with heart failure and iron deficiency. N Engl J Med 2009;361:2436.
17. Anand IS. Anemia and chronic heart failure implications and treatment options. J Am Coll Cardiol 2008;52:501.
18. Kalra PR, Collier T, Cowie MR, et al. Haemoglobin concentration and prognosis in new cases of heart failure. Lancet 2003;362:211.
19. Patel KV, Longo DL, Ershler WB, et al. Haemoglobin concentration and the risk of death in older adults: differences by race/ethnicity in the NHANES III follow-up. Br J Haematol 2009;145:514.
20. Felker GM, Shaw LK, Stough WG, et al. Anemia in patients with heart failure and preserved systolic function. Am Heart J 2006;151:457.

21. O'Meara E, Clayton T, McEntegart MB, et al. Clinical correlates and consequences of anemia in a broad spectrum of patients with heart failure: results of the Candesartan in Heart Failure: Assessment of Reduction in Mortality and Morbidity (CHARM) Program. Circulation 2006;113:986.

22. Nair D, Shlipak MG, Angeja B, et al. Association of anemia with diastolic dysfunction among patients with coronary artery disease in the Heart and Soul Study. Am J Cardiol 2005;95:332.

23. Anand I, McMurray JJ, Whitmore J, et al. Anemia and its relationship to clinical outcome in heart failure. Circulation 2004;110:149.

24. Windram JD, Loh PH, Rigby AS, et al. Relationship of high-sensitivity C-reactive protein to prognosis and other prognostic markers in outpatients with heart failure. Am Heart J 2007;153:1048.

25. Iversen PO, Andersson KB, Finsen AV, et al. Separate mechanisms cause anemia in ischemic versus non-ischemic murine heart failure. Am J Physiol Regul Integr Comp Physiol 2010;298(3): R808–14.

26. Adams KF Jr, Pina IL, Ghali JK, et al. Prospective evaluation of the association between hemoglobin concentration and quality of life in patients with heart failure. Am Heart J 2009;158:965.

27. Groenveld HF, Januzzi JL, Damman K, et al. Anemia and mortality in heart failure patients a systematic review and meta-analysis. J Am Coll Cardiol 2008; 52:818.

28. Horwich TB, Fonarow GC, Hamilton MA, et al. Anemia is associated with worse symptoms, greater impairment in functional capacity and a significant increase in mortality in patients with advanced heart failure. J Am Coll Cardiol 2002;39:1780.

29. Kosiborod M, Smith GL, Radford MJ, et al. The prognostic importance of anemia in patients with heart failure. Am J Med 2003;114:112.

30. Kosiborod M, Curtis JP, Wang Y, et al. Anemia and outcomes in patients with heart failure: a study from the National Heart Care Project. Arch Intern Med 2005;165:2237.

31. Peterson PN, Magid DJ, Lyons EE, et al. Association of longitudinal measures of hemoglobin and outcomes after hospitalization for heart failure. Am Heart J 2010;159:81.

32. Khan W, Deepak SM, Coppinger T, et al. Beta blocker treatment is associated with improvement in renal function and anaemia in patients with heart failure. Heart 1856;92:2006.

33. Albitar S, Genin R, Fen-Chong M, et al. High dose enalapril impairs the response to erythropoietin treatment in haemodialysis patients. Nephrol Dial Transplant 1998;13:1206.

34. Mohanram A, Zhang Z, Shahinfar S, et al. The effect of losartan on hemoglobin concentration and renal outcome in diabetic nephropathy of type 2 diabetes. Kidney Int 2008;73:630.

35. Schiffl H, Lang SM. Angiotensin-converting enzyme inhibitors but not angiotensin II AT 1 receptor antagonists affect erythropoiesis in patients with anemia of end-stage renal disease. Nephron 1999;81:106.

36. Sharma R, Francis DP, Pitt B, et al. Haemoglobin predicts survival in patients with chronic heart failure: a substudy of the ELITE II trial. Eur Heart J 2004;25:1021.

37. Cleland JG, Swedberg K, Follath F, et al. The Euro-Heart Failure survey programme—a survey on the quality of care among patients with heart failure in Europe. Part 1: patient characteristics and diagnosis. Eur Heart J 2003;24:442.

38. Herzog CA, Muster HA, Li S, et al. Impact of congestive heart failure, chronic kidney disease, and anemia on survival in the Medicare population. J Card Fail 2004;10:467.

39. Felker GM, Gattis WA, Leimberger JD, et al. Usefulness of anemia as a predictor of death and rehospitalization in patients with decompensated heart failure. Am J Cardiol 2003;92:625.

Pathophysiology of Anemia in Heart Failure

Inder S. Anand, MD, FRCP, DPhil (Oxon)

KEYWORDS

- Anemia • Heart failure • Erythropoietin
- High output heart failure • Chronic kidney
- Pathophysiology

Anemia is common in patients with acute and chronic systolic heart Failure (HF), and in HF with preserved ejection fraction, and may be present in nearly half the patients, depending on the definition of anemia used and on the population studied.[1,2] Anemia and lower or declining hemoglobin (Hgb) concentrations are powerful independent predictors of adverse outcomes in HF.[3–12] Correction of anemia may be useful in improving HF outcomes and may be a novel therapeutic target in HF. Early studies and meta-analyses have suggested that correction of anemia in patients with HF may improve signs, symptoms, left ventricular function, and quality of life.[13–18] However, given the real concerns about cardiovascular safety of higher Hgb with the use of erythropoietin stimulating agents (ESA) in patients with chronic kidney disease (CKD),[19–22] clinicians may not have the equipoise to treat anemia until the results of reduction of events with darbepoetin alfa in heart Failure, the large mortality and morbidity trial of the ESA darbepoetin in HF, are known.[23] Despite the increasing importance of anemia in HF, little is known about the pathogenesis of anemia in HF and the mechanisms by which anemia may worsen HF.[24]

In this article, the factors that are associated with the development and worsening of anemia in HF are discussed, and the possible mechanisms that may worsen HF in patients with anemia are examined.

WHO ARE THE PATIENTS WITH ANEMIA AND HEART FAILURE?

As compared to patients with HF who do not have anemia, patients who are anemic are more likely to be older, have diabetes, and CKD. These patients are also more likely to have worse HF as indicated by higher New York Heart Association (NYHA) class, lower exercise capacity, worse quality-of-life scores, greater peripheral edema, lower blood pressure, higher use of a diuretic and other cardiovascular medications, and worse neurohormonal and inflammatory profile.[1,7–10,25–27] Renal dysfunction, diabetes, peripheral edema, high brain natriuretic peptide (BNP) and C-reactive protein (CRP), low serum albumen, low weight, and low diastolic blood pressure were found to be independently associated with the likelihood of anemia in the Valsartan Heart Failure Trial (Val-HeFT) database.[10] Importantly, anemia does not seem to be related to left ventricular (LV) dysfunction and in the few studies where LV function measurements are available, Hgb was found to be inversely related to ejection fraction (EF); patients with lower Hgb had higher EF.[6,10,28] Moreover, spontaneous increase in Hgb over time may be associated with a decrease in LVEF,[10] and raising Hgb in patients with CKD has been shown to be associated with decrease in LVEF in a dose-dependent manner.[29]

POTENTIAL CAUSES OF ANEMIA DURING HEART FAILURE
Hematinic Abnormalities

Serum vitamin B12 and folic acid levels are low in only a minority of anemic patients with HF.[30,31] Gastrointestinal function is often abnormal in patients with HF[32] and this can lead to malabsorption causing iron and other nutritional

Heart Failure Program, VA Medical Center, 1, Veterans Drive, Minneapolis, MN 55417, USA
E-mail address: anand001@umn.edu

Heart Failure Clin 6 (2010) 279–288
doi:10.1016/j.hfc.2010.03.002
1551-7136/10/$ – see front matter. Published by Elsevier Inc.

heartfailure.theclinics.com

deficiencies.[33] Moreover, aspirin-induced gastrointestinal bleeding could also cause iron deficiency. Detailed investigations of iron homeostasis in anemic patients with HF are not available. Lacking standard criteria (ie, transferrin saturation [Tsat]; soluble transferrin receptor [sTFR]; or ferritin levels), the reported prevalence of iron deficiency has varied greatly from 5% to 21%.[25,30,31,34,35] In one study of anemic subjects with HF, 43% had either low serum iron (<8 µmol/L) or ferritin (<30 µg/L), but microcytic anemia was seen in only 6% of subjects.[36] In contrast, Nanas and colleagues[37] found depleted iron stores in the bone marrow of 73% subjects despite normal serum iron, ferritin, and erythropoietin. The mean corpuscular volume was at the lower limit of normal suggesting that microcytic anemia was not present in all subjects. These findings might be explained by diversion of iron from the bone marrow to the other reticuloendothelial stores where it is not available for erythropoiesis even though serum iron and ferritin are normal or increased, a feature of anemia of chronic disease.[38] Therefore, either an absolute or relative iron deficiency may be more common than previously thought.

Chronic Kidney Disease and Impaired Erythropoietin Production

Erythropoietin is a glycoprotein hormone that regulates erythroid cell proliferation in the bone marrow in response to tissue hypoxia. Erythropoietin is produced primarily in the kidney by specialized peritubular fibroblasts that are situated within the cortex and outer medulla.[39–41] The primary stimulus for erythropoietin production is reduced oxygen tension at the level of the peritubular fibroblasts where oxygen sensing is considered to occur. Low PO_2 activates hypoxia-inducible factor-1 (HIF-1), which in turn induces transcription of the erythropoietin gene.[42] The kidney is susceptible to hypoxia despite the fact that it receives nearly 25% of the cardiac output and uses less that 10% of the oxygen delivered, which is because oxygen tension is remarkably inhomogeneous across the renal parenchyma. To maintain the osmotic gradient generated by the loop of Henle, the arterial and venous blood vessels supplying it run countercurrent and in close contact. This leads to shunt diffusion of oxygen between the arterial and venous circulation, causing an oxygen gradient across the renal parenchyma.[40] Consequently, oxygen tension decreases with increasing distance from the surface of the kidney, reaching around 10 mmHg at the tips of the cortical pyramids where the oxygen sensing and erythropoietin producing cells

are located. This remarkable design makes this area sensitive to small changes in the oxygen tension resulting from the imbalance between oxygen delivery and utilization. Oxygen delivery to this region is determined by renal blood flow (RBF), hematocrit, and the P_{50} of the hemoglobin oxygen-dissociation curve. Conversely, oxygen consumption is determined by proximal tubular sodium reabsorption, which is largely dependent on the glomerular filtration rate (GFR).

Although there is extensive evidence for inadequate erythropoietin production in CKD, the mechanisms remain unclear. Tubulointerstitial fibrosis, tubular loss, and vascular obliteration are probably the most important factors that contribute to a decrease in erythropoietin-producing cells.[43] In HF, the RBF is decreased[44] and approximately 50% of patients with HF have some renal dysfunction.[45–47] These findings lead to the suggestion that decreased renal erythropoietin production is the cause of anemia in HF. Only a few studies have examined the relation between RBF and erythropoietin in subjects with HF. Two small studies found that RBF was an independent determinant of erythropoietin secretion,[48,49] but a more recent study could not confirm these findings[50] in a larger subset of subjects with HF. However, erythropoietin levels are not always low and are often increased, in proportion to the severity of HF but lower than expected for the degree of anemia, and do not correlate with the Hgb level, suggesting a blunted erythropoietin response.[25,51–55] Belonje and colleagues[54] have recently reported erythropoietin levels in 605 subjects with HF randomized in the coordinating study evaluating outcomes of advising and counseling in heart failure trial. They found that erythropoietin levels were lower than expected in the majority of subjects (79%), whereas, 12% of subjects had levels as expected and 9% has erythropoietin levels higher than expected. High levels of erythropoietin at baseline and 6 months, as well as higher observed to predicted ratio of erythropoietin to Hgb level were independently related to increased risk for mortality.[54] The relation between RBF and erythropoietin production may be more complex because many other factors affect erythropoietin production in HF (**Fig. 1**). High levels of angiotensin II (Ang II) seen in HF reduce oxygen supply by decreasing RBF. At the same time, an Ang II-induced decrease in GFR causes an increase in proximal tubular sodium reabsorption that increases oxygen demand. These factors stimulate erythropoietin production by reducing oxygen delivery at the level of the erythropoietin-producing cells. Several factors might explain the finding that

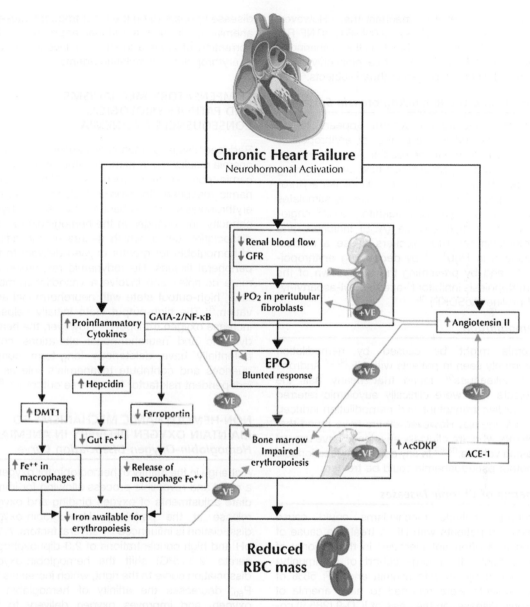

Fig. 1. Possible mechanisms involved in the genesis of anemia in heart failure. ACE-I, angiotensin converting enzyme inhibitor; AcSDKP, N-acetyl-seryl-aspartyl-lysyl-proline; ARB, angiotensin receptor blocker; DMT1, Divalent metal transporter 1. (*Reproduced from* Anand IS. Anemia and chronic heart failure: Implications and treatment options. J Am Coll Cardiol 2008;52(7):501–11; with permission.)

erythropoietin response is blunted and the levels are inappropriately low to the degree of anemia in HF. Perhaps the most important factor is the role played by inflammation. Tumor necrosis factor-α (TNF-α) and its soluble receptors (sTNF-R1 and sTNF-R2); interleukin-6 (IL-6) and several other proinflammatory cytokines[25,56]; circulating neutrophils; and CRP are increased in patients with HF[57] and are inversely related to hemoglobin.[26,58] IL-6 and TNF-α inhibit erythropoietin production in the kidney by activating GATA-2

and NF-κB.[59] Therefore, erythropoietin levels may be lower than expected. In addition, these cytokines also directly inhibit the differentiation and proliferation of erythroid progenitor cells in the bone marrow.[60,61] Moreover, IL-6 stimulates the production of the acute phase protein hepcidin from the liver that inhibits the duodenal absorption of iron.[32] Furthermore, IL-6 downregulates the expression of ferroportin, preventing the release of iron from body stores.[62] Thus, proinflammatory cytokines may contribute to the development of anemia by several mechanisms. However, elevated levels of TNF-α, sTNF-R1, sTNF-R2, and IL-6 in the anemic subjects in the Vesnarinone Heart Failure Trial (VEST) could explain only 5% of the variability in Hgb seen in those subjects.[26]

Anemia and the Renin-Angiotensin System

The renin-angiotensin system appears to be closely involved in the control of erythropoiesis (see **Fig. 1**). As mentioned earlier, Ang II decreases PO_2 by reducing renal blood flow and increasing oxygen demand, and thereby stimulates erythropoietin production. Ang II also directly stimulates bone marrow erythroid progenitor cells.[63] Angiotensin converting enzyme (ACE) inhibitors and angiotensin receptor blockers cause a modest reduction in Hgb[10,64] by decreasing erythropoietin,[65] and by preventing the breakdown of the hematopoiesis inhibitor N-acetyl-seryl-aspartyl-lysyl-proline (AcSDKP).[66]

Hemodilution

Anemia might be caused by hemodilution commonly seen in patients with HF.[50,67] Androne and colleagues[67] found that nearly half the subjects who were clinically euvolemic referred for cardiac transplant had hemodilution-induced pseudoanemia. However, others have found that patients who are clinically euvolemic have normal plasma volume.[68,69] In any case, it is questionable whether pseudoanemia could be treated.

Anemia of Chronic Diseases

Although multiple mechanisms could cause anemia in patients with HF, a treatable cause of anemia is often not identified in the majority of the patients. In a large cohort of community-dwelling subjects with anemia and HF, 58% of the subjects were reported to have anemia of chronic disease, on the basis of ICD-9 (285.9) codes alone,[34] although evidence supporting the presence of anemia of chronic disease was not available in that study. Opasich and colleagues[25] do provided conclusive evidence of the existence of anemia of chronic disease in HF. These authors studied 148 well-characterized subjects with stable HF and anemia. A specific cause of anemia including CKD, iron, folic acid, vitamin B12 deficiency, and β-thalassemia could be identified in only 43% of the cases. Iron deficiency was seen in only 5% of the subjects. In the vast majority of the remaining subjects (57%), they found proinflammatory cytokine activation, inadequate erythropoietin production, or defective iron utilization despite adequate iron stores, suggesting anemia of chronic disease.[38] Therefore, anemia of chronic

disease appears to be the most frequent cause of anemia in HF and a rational approach to the correction of anemia in HF may involve the use of erythropoiesis-stimulating agents.

COMPENSATORY MECHANISMS AND PATHOPHYSIOLOGICAL CONSEQUENCES OF ANEMIA

Reduced tissue oxygenation caused by chronic anemia results in non-hemodynamic and hemodynamic compensatory responses. Non-hemodynamic responses to hypoxia include increase in erythropoiesis to enhance oxygen carrying capacity and changes in the hemoglobin-oxygen dissociation curve, which decreases the affinity of hemoglobin for greater oxygen delivery to the peripheral tissues. Hemodynamic responses are more complex and involve a vasodilation-mediated, high-output state with neurohormonal activation.[70] The high-output state initially helps to increase oxygen transport.[71] However, the hemodynamic and neurohormonal alterations could potentially have deleterious long-term consequences and contribute to anemia's role as an independent risk factor for adverse outcomes.[3–10]

NON-HEMODYNAMIC MECHANISMS TO MAINTAIN OXYGEN DELIVERY IN ANEMIA
Hemoglobin-Oxygen Dissociation Curve

A change in the affinity of hemoglobin for oxygen is a rapid and reversible process allowing for immediate adjustments of oxygen binding and oxygen release at the periphery. Hemoglobin-oxygen dissociation is influenced by several factors. A low pH and high concentrations of 2,3-diphosphoglycerate (2,3-DPG) shift the hemoglobin-oxygen dissociation curve to the right, which increases the P_{50}, decreases the affinity of hemoglobin for oxygen, and improves oxygen delivery to the tissues. In chronic anemia the red blood cell (RBC) concentration of 2,3-DPG is increased and the hemoglobin-oxygen dissociation curve is shifted to the right.[72,73] A right-shifted curve is the least energy-consuming mechanism to support increased oxygen delivery to the tissues without a significant increase in cardiac output. The 2,3-diphosphoglycerate is a metabolic intermediate of RBC glycolysis and is quantitatively the most important organic phosphate regulating oxygen affinity in erythrocytes.[74] The activity of many red blood cell glycolytic enzymes, and therefore the concentrations of 2,3-DPG and adenosine triphosphate, are largely dependent on the age of the erythrocyte. Enzyme activity is especially high in young red blood cells and decreases with increasing cell age.

Consequently, young erythrocytes have a right-shifted oxygen dissociation curve and a steeper curve slope, which further adds to the effectiveness of oxygen unloading.[75]

HEMODYNAMIC MECHANISMS TO MAINTAIN OXYGEN DELIVERY IN ANEMIA

Because erythropoiesis is defective in HF, compensatory hemodynamic responses may predominate. In chronic severe anemia, low Hgb reduces systemic vascular resistance (SVR)[70,76] caused by decreases in blood viscosity and enhanced nitric oxide-mediated vasodilation.[76,77] Low SVR reduces blood pressure and causes baroreceptor-mediated neurohormonal activation,[70] identical to that seen in low output HF.[44,78] The increased sympathetic and renin-angiotensin activity decreases RBF and GFR, resulting in salt and water retention by the kidneys and expansion of the extracellular and plasma volumes, and may result in the clinical syndrome of HF. In animal models of anemia, increased hemodynamic load and chronic elevation of catecholamines and Ang II causes LV hypertrophy, increase in LV mass, and LV dilation,[79–81] which may have deleterious long-term consequences. However, the combined effect of volume expansion and vasodilation increases

the cardiac output,[70] which may help to increase oxygen transport.[71] Correction of anemia in patients with normal LV function causes a rapid and complete regression of the syndrome of high output HF.[70,76] It should be emphasized that these hemodynamic and neurohormonal responses were observed in patients with chronic severe anemia. It is unclear whether these mechanisms are also operative in patients with HF with less severe anemia. However, similar hemodynamic changes have also been reported in patients with CKD who have mild to moderate anemia. McMahon and colleagues[29] found that in subjects with CKD, when Hgb was increased progressively from 8.5 to 10 to 14 g/dL with epoetin, the cardiac output (7.0 to 6.6 to 5.2 L/min) and the fractional shortening (36% to 33% to 29%) decreased significantly. Therefore, these data suggest that correction of anemia is unlikely to improve EF. The possible sequence of events in the pathogenesis of HF in anemia is shown in **Fig. 2**.

POSSIBLE MECHANISMS TO EXPLAIN THE POOR OUTCOMES IN ANEMIA AND HEART FAILURE

Anemia and low Hgb are independently associated with increased risk for mortality in acute

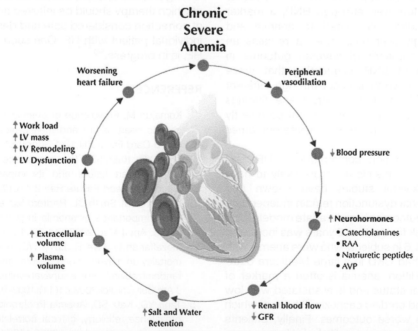

Fig. 2. The possible sequence of events involved in the pathogenesis of heart failure in chronic severe anemia. AVP, arginine vasopressin; GFR, glomerular filtration rate; RAA, renin-angiotensin-aldosterone. (*Reproduced from* Anand IS. Anemia and chronic heart failure: implications and treatment options. J Am Coll Cardiol 2008;52(7):501–11; with permission.)

and chronic HF with impaired[3,4,6–10,34,82,83] and preserved LV function.[6,83–86] Anemia increased the risk for death in these studies by 20% to 50%. The mechanisms linking anemia to increased mortality and morbidity are not entirely clear, but are likely to be complex and multifactorial. Increased myocardial workload to compensate for reduced tissue oxygen delivery and volume overload can lead to unfavorable LV remodeling with LV hypertrophy and dilation that may contribute to adverse outcomes.[87] Although LV hypertrophy is consistently seen in patients who have CKD with anemia,[88] it is unclear whether it is related to anemia or the associated hypertension.[89] Treatment of anemia with erythropoiesis stimulating agents has, however, not shown to reverse LV hypertrophy in several clinical trials,[90–92] which may be related to the development of irreversible myocardial fibrosis.[93] There are no clinical data linking LV hypertrophy and anemia in HF and it is not known whether correction of anemia in HF reverses LV hypertrophy. However, in a substudy on subjects with HF enrolled in the randomized etanercept North American strategy to study antagonism of cytokines (RENAISSANCE) trial, a 1-g/dL spontaneous increase in Hgb over a period of 24 weeks was associated with a 4.1-g/m^2 decrease in LV mass.[9] As mentioned earlier, patients with lower Hgb tend to have a higher LVEF.[6,10,28] Moreover, although BNP, a marker of LV dysfunction, is related to anemia and change in Hgb over time, anemia remains an independent predictor of adverse outcome in the presence of BNP, suggesting that these variables may have their effect through different mechanisms.[10] Taken together, these findings suggest that LV dysfunction may not be directly involved in the pathogenesis of worse outcomes in anemia.

CKD is a common comorbidity in HF, and patients who are anemic are more likely to have CKD.[8,46,94] Several studies have shown that anemia and renal dysfunction remain independent predictors of outcomes in multivariate models.[6,8,10] The relative risk for death at 2 years was increased by a factor of 1.6 in subjects who were anemic with HF who also had CKD in a large Medicare database.[95] In addition, anemia is often a marker of poor nutritional status and is associated with low albumin[6,10] and cardiac cachexia,[96] both of which are related to worse outcomes. Finally, patients who are anemic are more likely to have worse neurohormonal and proinflammatory cytokine profile, which may also contribute to worse outcomes.[26,58] Thus, anemia may be related to a worse prognosis through multiple and overlapping mechanisms.

SUMMARY

In conclusion, although the mechanisms involved in the genesis of anemia in HF are not entirely clear, the weight of the evidence suggests that renal dysfunction, and neurohormonal and proinflammatory cytokine activation favors the development of anemia of chronic disease. Likewise, the mechanisms by which anemia worsens HF outcomes are also unknown. Increased myocardial workload associated with anemia can lead to LV hypertrophy and LV dilation. In patients with normal LV function, severe anemia leads to a vasodilation-mediated, high-output state with fluid retention that rapidly reverses with the correction of anemia. Because increase in Hgb is associated with an elevation in the systemic vascular resistance, it is unlikely that correction of anemia will improve impaired LV function, and there are no data to show the LV hypertrophy regresses on increasing Hgb in patients with HF. However, uncontrolled studies have shown beneficial effects of treating anemia in patients with HF.[13,15,97] Further studies are therefore required to understand the basis of the remarkable association of anemia with HF mortality and morbidity, to prospectively assess the potential benefit of correcting anemia, and to evaluate the ideal threshold at which therapy should be initiated and the extent of correction considered safe and desirable in the individual patient with HF. One such study, RED-HF, is in progress.[98]

REFERENCES

1. Komajda M. Prevalence of anemia in patients with chronic heart failure and their clinical characteristics. J Card Fail 2004;10(1 Suppl):S1–4.
2. Tang YD, Katz SD. The prevalence of anemia in chronic heart failure and its impact on clinical outcomes. Heart Failure Rev 2008;13(4):387–92.
3. Kosiborod M, Smith GL, Radford MJ, et al. The prognostic importance of anemia in patients with heart failure. Am J Med 2003;114(2):112–9.
4. Mozaffarian D, Nye R, Levy WC. Anemia predicts mortality in severe heart failure: the prospective randomized amlodipine survival evaluation (PRAISE). J Am Coll Cardiol 2003;41(11):1933–9.
5. Tang YD, Katz SD. Anemia in chronic heart failure: prevalence, etiology, clinical correlates, and treatment options. Circulation 2006;113(20):2454–61.
6. O'Meara E, Clayton T, McEntegart MB, et al. Clinical correlates and consequences of anemia in a broad spectrum of patients with heart failure: results of

the candesartan in Heart Failure: Assessment of Reduction in Mortality and Morbidity (CHARM) Program. Circulation 2006;113(7):986–94.

7. Horwich TB, Fonarow GC, Hamilton MA, et al. Anemia is associated with worse symptoms, greater impairment in functional capacity and a significant increase in mortality in patients with advanced heart failure. J Am Coll Cardiol 2002;39(11):1780–6.

8. Al-Ahmad A, Rand WM, Manjunath G, et al. Reduced kidney function and anemia as risk factors for mortality in patients with left ventricular dysfunction. J Am Coll Cardiol 2001;38(4):955–62.

9. Anand I, McMurray JJ, Whitmore J, et al. Anemia and its relationship to clinical outcome in heart failure. Circulation 2004;110(2):149–54.

10. Anand IS, Kuskowski MA, Rector TS, et al. Anemia and change in hemoglobin over time related to mortality and morbidity in patients with chronic heart failure: results from Val-HeFT. Circulation 2005;112(8):1121–7.

11. Anand IS. Anemia and chronic heart failure implications and treatment options. J Am Coll Cardiol 2008;52(7):501–11.

12. Peterson PN, Magid DJ, Lyons EE, et al. Association of longitudinal measures of hemoglobin and outcomes after hospitalization for heart failure. Am Heart J 2010;159(1):81–9.

13. Silverberg DS, Wexler D, Blum M, et al. The use of subcutaneous erythropoietin and intravenous iron for the treatment of the anemia of severe, resistant congestive heart failure improves cardiac and renal function and functional cardiac class, and markedly reduces hospitalizations. J Am Coll Cardiol 2000;35(7):1737–44.

14. Silverberg DS, Wexler D, Sheps D, et al. The effect of correction of mild anemia in severe, resistant congestive heart failure using subcutaneous erythropoietin and intravenous iron: a randomized controlled study. J Am Coll Cardiol 2001;37(7):1775–80.

15. Mancini DM, Katz SD, Lang CC, et al. Effect of erythropoietin on exercise capacity in patients with moderate to severe chronic heart failure. Circulation 2003;107(2):294–9.

16. Palazzuoli A, Silverberg DS, Iovine F, et al. Effects of beta-erythropoietin treatment on left ventricular remodeling, systolic function, and B-type natriuretic peptide levels in patients with the cardiorenal anemia syndrome. Am Heart J 2007;154(4):645, e9–15.

17. Ghali JK, Anand IS, Abraham WT, et al. Randomized double-blind trial of darbepoetin alfa in patients with symptomatic heart failure and anemia. Circulation 2008;117:526–35.

18. van der Meer P, Groenveld HF, Januzzi JL Jr, et al. Erythropoietin treatment in patients with chronic heart failure: a meta-analysis. Heart 2009;95(16):1309–14.

19. Besarab A, Bolton WK, Browne JK, et al. The effects of normal as compared with low hematocrit values in patients with cardiac disease who are receiving hemodialysis and epoetin. N Engl J Med 1998;339(9):584–90.

20. Singh AK, Szczech L, Tang KL, et al. Correction of anemia with epoetin alfa in chronic kidney disease. N Engl J Med 2006;355(20):2085–98.

21. Drueke TB, Locatelli F, Clyne N, et al. Normalization of hemoglobin level in patients with chronic kidney disease and anemia. N Engl J Med 2006;355(20):2071–84.

22. Pfeffer MA, Burdmann EA, Chen CY, et al. A trial of darbepoetin alfa in type 2 diabetes and chronic kidney disease. N Engl J Med 2009;361(21):2019–32.

23. McMurray JJ, Anand IS, Diaz R, et al. Design of the reduction of events with darbepoetin alfa in heart failure (RED-HF): a phase III, anaemia correction, morbidity-mortality trial. Eur J Heart Fail 2009;11(8):795–801.

24. Anand IS. Heart failure and anemia: mechanisms and pathophysiology. Heart Fail Rev 2008;13(4):379–86.

25. Opasich C, Cazzola M, Scelsi L, et al. Blunted erythropoietin production and defective iron supply for erythropoiesis as major causes of anaemia in patients with chronic heart failure. Eur Heart J 2005;26(21):2232–7.

26. Anand IS, Rector I, Deswal A, et al. Relationship between proinflammatory cytokines and anemia in heart failure. Eur Heart J 2006,27(Suppl 1):485.

27. Maggioni AP, Opasich C, Anand I, et al. Anemia in patients with heart failure: prevalence and prognostic role in a controlled trial and in clinical practice. J Card Fail 2005;11(2):91–8.

28. Philipp S, Ollmann H, Schink T, et al. The impact of anaemia and kidney function in congestive heart failure and preserved systolic function. Nephrol Dial Transplant 2005;20(5):915–9.

29. McMahon LP, Mason K, Skinner SL, et al. Effects of haemoglobin normalization on quality of life and cardiovascular parameters in end-stage renal failure. Nephrol Dial Transplant 2000;15(9):1425–30.

30. Witte KK, Desilva R, Chattopadhyay S, et al. Are hematinic deficiencies the cause of anemia in chronic heart failure? Am Heart J 2004;147(5):924–30.

31. Cromie N, Lee C, Struthers AD. Anaemia in chronic heart failure: what is its frequency in the UK and its underlying causes? Heart 2002;87(4):377–8.

32. Sandek A, Bauditz J, Swidsinski A, et al. Altered intestinal function in patients with chronic heart failure. J Am Coll Cardiol 2007;50(16):1561–9.

33. Anker SD, Chua TP, Ponikowski P, et al. Hormonal changes and catabolic/anabolic imbalance in chronic heart failure and their importance for cardiac cachexia. Circulation 1997;96(2):526–34.

34. Ezekowitz JA, McAlister FA, Armstrong PW. Anemia is common in heart failure and is associated with

poor outcomes: insights from a cohort of 12 065 patients with new-onset heart failure. Circulation 2003;107(2):223–5.

35. Felker GM, Gattis WA, Leimberger JD, et al. Usefulness of anemia as a predictor of death and rehospitalization in patients with decompensated heart failure. Am J Cardiol 2003;92(5):625–8.

36. de Silva R, Rigby AS, Witte KK, et al. Anemia, renal dysfunction, and their interaction in patients with chronic heart failure. Am J Cardiol 2006;98(3):391–8.

37. Nanas JN, Matsouka C, Karageorgopoulos D, et al. Etiology of anemia in patients with advanced heart failure. J Am Coll Cardiol 2006;48(12):2485–9.

38. Weiss G, Goodnough LT. Anemia of chronic disease. N Engl J Med 2005;352(10):1011–23.

39. Eckardt KU, Koury ST, Tan CC, et al. Distribution of erythropoietin producing cells in rat kidneys during hypoxic hypoxia. Kidney Int 1993;43(4):815–23.

40. Bauer C, Kurtz A. Oxygen sensing in the kidney and its relation to erythropoietin production. Annu Rev Physiol 1989;51:845–56.

41. Bachmann S, Le Hir M, Eckardt KU. Co-localization of erythropoietin mRNA and ecto-5'-nucleotidase immunoreactivity in peritubular cells of rat renal cortex indicates that fibroblasts produce erythropoietin. J Histochem Cytochem 1993;41(3):335–41.

42. Mole DR, Ratcliffe PJ. Cellular oxygen sensing in health and disease. Pediatr Nephrol 2008;23(5):681–94.

43. Nangaku M. Chronic hypoxia and tubulointerstitial injury: a final common pathway to end-stage renal failure. J Am Soc Nephrol 2006;17(1):17–25.

44. Anand IS, Ferrari R, Kalra GS, et al. Edema of cardiac origin. Studies of body water and sodium, renal function, hemodynamic indexes, and plasma hormones in untreated congestive cardiac failure. Circulation 1989;80(2):299–305.

45. McCullough PA, Lepor NE. Piecing together the evidence on anemia: the link between chronic kidney disease and cardiovascular disease. Rev Cardiovasc Med 2005;6(Suppl 3):S4–12.

46. Anand IS. Pathogenesis of anemia in cardiorenal disease. Rev Cardiovasc Med 2005;6(Suppl 3):S13–21.

47. McClellan WM, Flanders WD, Langston RD, et al. Anemia and renal insufficiency are independent risk factors for death among patients with congestive heart failure admitted to community hospitals: a population-based study. J Am Soc Nephrol 2002;13(7):1928–36.

48. Jensen JD, Eiskjaer H, Bagger JP, et al. Elevated level of erythropoietin in congestive heart failure relationship to renal perfusion and plasma renin. J Intern Med 1993;233(2):125–30.

49. Pham I, Andrivet P, Sediame S, et al. Increased erythropoietin synthesis in patients with COLD or left heart failure is related to alterations in renal haemodynamics. Eur J Clin Invest 2001;31(2):103–9.

50. Westenbrink BD, Visser FW, Voors AA, et al. Anaemia in chronic heart failure is not only related to impaired renal perfusion and blunted erythropoietin production, but to fluid retention as well. Eur Heart J 2007;28(2):166–71.

51. Volpe M, Tritto C, Testa U, et al. Blood levels of erythropoietin in congestive heart failure and correlation with clinical, hemodynamic, and hormonal profiles. Am J Cardiol 1994;74(5):468–73.

52. George J, Patal S, Wexler D, et al. Circulating erythropoietin levels and prognosis in patients with congestive heart failure: comparison with neurohormonal and inflammatory markers. Arch Intern Med 2005;165(11):1304–9.

53. van der Meer P, Voors AA, Lipsic E, et al. Prognostic value of plasma erythropoietin on mortality in patients with chronic heart failure. J Am Coll Cardiol 2004;44(1):63–7.

54. Belonje AM, Voors AA, van der Meer P, et al. Endogenous erythropoietin and outcome in heart failure. Circulation 2010;121(2):245–51.

55. Belonje AM, Westenbrink BD, Voors AA, et al. Erythropoietin levels in heart failure after an acute myocardial infarction: determinants, prognostic value, and the effects of captopril versus losartan. Am Heart J 2009;157(1):91–6.

56. Deswal A, Petersen NJ, Feldman AM, et al. Cytokines and cytokine receptors in advanced heart failure: an analysis of the cytokine database from the Vesnarinone trial (VEST). Circulation 2001;103(16):2055–9.

57. Anand IS, Latini R, Florea VG, et al. C-reactive protein in heart failure: prognostic value and the effect of valsartan. Circulation 2005;112(10):1428–34.

58. Rauchhaus M, Koloczek V, Volk H, et al. Inflammatory cytokines and the possible immunological role for lipoproteins in chronic heart failure. Int J Cardiol 2000;76(2–3):125–33.

59. Jelkmann W. Proinflammatory cytokines lowering erythropoietin production. J Interferon Cytokine Res 1998;18(8):555–9.

60. Means RT Jr. Recent developments in the anemia of chronic disease. Curr Hematol Rep 2003;2(2):116–21.

61. Macdougall IC, Cooper AC. Erythropoietin resistance: the role of inflammation and pro-inflammatory cytokines. Nephrol Dial Transplant 2002;17(Suppl 11):39–43.

62. Nemeth E, Rivera S, Gabayan V, et al. IL-6 mediates hypoferremia of inflammation by inducing the synthesis of the iron regulatory hormone hepcidin. J Clin Invest 2004;113(9):1271–6.

63. Mrug M, Stopka T, Julian BA, et al. Angiotensin II stimulates proliferation of normal early erythroid progenitors. J Clin Invest 1997;100(9):2310–4.

64. Albitar S, Genin R, Fen-Chong M, et al. High dose enalapril impairs the response to erythropoietin treatment in haemodialysis patients. Nephrol Dial Transplant 1998;13(5):1206–10.
65. Fyhrquist F, Karppinen K, Honkanen T, et al. High serum erythropoietin levels are normalized during treatment of congestive heart failure with enalapril. J Intern Med 1989;226(4):257–60.
66. van der Meer P, Lipsic E, Westenbrink BD, et al. Levels of hematopoiesis inhibitor N-acetyl-seryl-aspartyl-lysyl-proline partially explain the occurrence of anemia in heart failure. Circulation 2005;112(12):1743–7.
67. Androne AS, Katz SD, Lund L, et al. Hemodilution is common in patients with advanced heart failure. Circulation 2003;107(2):226–9.
68. Anand IS, Veall N, Kalra GS, et al. Treatment of heart failure with diuretics: body compartments, renal function and plasma hormones. Eur Heart J 1989;10(5):445–50.
69. Kalra PR, Anagnostopoulos C, Bolger AP, et al. The regulation and measurement of plasma volume in heart failure. J Am Coll Cardiol 2002;39(12):1901–8.
70. Anand IS, Chandrashekhar Y, Ferrari R, et al. Pathogenesis of oedema in chronic severe anaemia: studies of body water and sodium, renal function, haemodynamic variables, and plasma hormones. Br Heart J 1993;70(4):357–62.
71. Varat MA, Adolph RJ, Fowler NO. Cardiovascular effects of anemia. Am Heart J 1972;83(3):415–26.
72. Oski FA, Marshall BE, Cohen PJ, et al. The role of the left-shifted or right-shifted oxygen-hemoglobin equilibrium curve. Ann Intern Med 1971;74(1):44–6.
73. Metivier F, Marchais SJ, Guerin AP, et al. Pathophysiology of anaemia: focus on the heart and blood vessels. Nephrol Dial Transplant 2000;15(Suppl 3):14–8.
74. Brewer GJ. 2,3-DPG and erythrocyte oxygen affinity. Annu Rev Med 1974;25:29–38.
75. Schmidt W, Boning D, Braumann KM. Red cell age effects on metabolism and oxygen affinity in humans. Respir Physiol 1987;68(2):215–25.
76. Anand IS, Chandrashekhar Y, Wander GS, et al. Endothelium-derived relaxing factor is important in mediating the high output state in chronic severe anemia. J Am Coll Cardiol 1995;25(6):1402–7.
77. Ni Z, Morcos S, Vaziri ND. Up-regulation of renal and vascular nitric oxide synthase in iron-deficiency anemia. Kidney Int 1997;52(1):195–201.
78. Anand IS, Ferrari R, Kalra GS, et al. Pathogenesis of edema in constrictive pericarditis. Studies of body water and sodium, renal function, hemodynamics, and plasma hormones before and after pericardiectomy. Circulation 1991;83(6):1880–7.
79. Datta BN, Silver MD. Cardiomegaly in chronic anemia in rats and man experimental study including ultrastructural, histometric, and stereologic observations. Lab Invest 1975;32(4):503–14.
80. Olivetti G, Quaini F, Lagrasta C, et al. Myocyte cellular hypertrophy and hyperplasia contribute to ventricular wall remodeling in anemia-induced cardiac hypertrophy in rats. Am J Pathol 1992;141(1):227–39.
81. Rakusan K, Cicutti N, Kolar F. Effect of anemia on cardiac function, microvascular structure, and capillary hematocrit in rat hearts. Am J Physiol Heart Circ Physiol 2001;280(3):H1407–14.
82. Ishani A, Weinhandl E, Zhao Z, et al. Angiotensin-converting enzyme inhibitor as a risk factor for the development of anemia, and the impact of incident anemia on mortality in patients with left ventricular dysfunction. J Am Coll Cardiol 2005;45(3):391–9.
83. Go AS, Yang J, Ackerson LM, et al. Hemoglobin level, chronic kidney disease, and the risks of death and hospitalization in adults with chronic heart failure: the Anemia in Chronic Heart Failure: Outcomes and Resource Utilization (ANCHOR) Study. Circulation 2006;113(23):2713–23.
84. Berry C, Norrie J, Hogg K, et al. The prevalence, nature, and importance of hematologic abnormalities in heart failure. Am Heart J 2006;151(6):1313–21.
85. Felker GM, Shaw LK, Stough WG, et al. Anemia in patients with heart failure and preserved systolic function. Am Heart J 2006;151(2):457–62.
86. Brucks S, Little WC, Chao T, et al. Relation of anemia to diastolic heart failure and the effect on outcome. Am J Cardiol 2004;93(8):1055–7.
87. Lauer MS, Evans JC, Levy D. Prognostic implications of subclinical left ventricular dilatation and systolic dysfunction in men free of overt cardiovascular disease (the Framingham Heart Study). Am J Cardiol 1992;70(13):1180–4.
88. Levin A. Prevalence of cardiovascular damage in early renal disease. Nephrol Dial Transplant 2001;16(Suppl 2):7–11.
89. Levin A. Anemia and left ventricular hypertrophy in chronic kidney disease populations: a review of the current state of knowledge. Kidney Int Suppl 2002;80:35–8.
90. Parfrey PS, Foley RN, Wittreich BH, et al. Double-blind comparison of full and partial anemia correction in incident hemodialysis patients without symptomatic heart disease. J Am Soc Nephrol 2005;16(7):2180–9.
91. Roger SD, McMahon LP, Clarkson A, et al. Effects of early and late intervention with epoetin alpha on left ventricular mass among patients with chronic kidney disease (stage 3 or 4): results of a randomized clinical trial. J Am Soc Nephrol 2004;15(1):148–56.
92. Levin A. The treatment of anemia in chronic kidney disease: understandings in 2006. Curr Opin Nephrol Hypertens 2007;16(3):267–71.
93. Mall G, Huther W, Schneider J, et al. Diffuse intermyocardiocytic fibrosis in uraemic patients. Nephrol Dial Transplant 1990;5(1):39–44.

94. McCullough PA, Lepor NE. The deadly triangle of anemia, renal insufficiency, and cardiovascular disease: implications for prognosis and treatment. Rev Cardiovasc Med 2005;6(1):1–10.

95. Collins AJ. The hemoglobin link to adverse outcomes. Adv Stud Med 2003;3(3C):S194–7.

96. Anker SD, Coats AJ. Cardiac cachexia: a syndrome with impaired survival and immune and neuroendocrine activation. Chest 1999; 115(3):836–47.

97. Silverberg DS, Wexler D, Blum M, et al. The effect of correction of anaemia in diabetics and non-diabetics with severe resistant congestive heart failure and chronic renal failure by subcutaneous erythropoietin and intravenous iron. Nephrol Dial Transplant 2003; 18(1):141–6.

98. van Veldhuisen DJ, McMurray JJ. Are erythropoietin stimulating proteins safe and efficacious in heart failure? Why we need an adequately powered randomised outcome trial. Eur J Heart Fail 2007;9(2):110–2.

Mediators of Anemia in Chronic Heart Failure

Thierry H. Le Jemtel, MD*, Salman Arain, MD

KEYWORDS

- Chronic heart failure • Anemia
- Impaired iron metabolism • Inflammatory stress

Anemia has received much attention in patients with chronic heart failure (CHF) for 2 major reasons.[1,2] First, it is a highly prevalent condition in patients with CHF and, second, the presence of anemia predicts a poor clinical outcome independently from the presence of other comorbid conditions including chronic kidney disease (CKD).[3–7] The World Health Organization (WHO) defines anemia as a hemoglobin concentration below 12 g/dL in women and 13 g/dL in men.[8] According to this definition, the prevalence of anemia is extremely variable, ranging from 9% to 70% in CHF.[9,10] Several clinical characteristics are likely to account for such variability in the prevalence of anemia in CHF.[1] These clinical characteristics include increasing age, female gender, CKD, low body mass index (BMI), fluid accumulation, and clinical deterioration requiring hospitalization. Whereas anemia is well known to occur in patients with CHF, the precise mechanisms that mediate a fall in hemoglobin concentration and ultimately anemia have yet to be elucidated.[11,12] We first review the clinical characteristics of patients with CHF who are likely to present with anemia. The role of specific causes of anemia such as impaired iron metabolism, blunted erythropoietin production and response, renin-angiotensin system (RAS) activity, and the role of systemic inflammation are then discussed in the context of CHF. Overall, whereas the association of anemia and CHF has been unequivocally associated with a worse prognosis compared with CHF alone, the triggers and mechanisms that underlie this association remain often speculative and thus not yet amenable to specific therapy.[13]

CLINICAL CHARACTERISTICS ASSOCIATED WITH ANEMIA IN CHF

Age

Among community residents 85 years or older, 17% of women and 24% of men are anemic according to the WHO definition.[8] The 5-year mortality of anemic women and men is 1.6 and 2.4 times greater, respectively, compared with their nonanemic counterparts.[8] Of note, the mortality risk associated with anemia remains unchanged after adjustments are made for functional capacity and preexisting conditions.[8] Thus, independently from CHF, the presence of anemia has important prognostic implications in older patients. The poor prognosis of anemia with advancing age has special implications for CHF when one considers that the median age of patients with CHF is steadily increasing, particularly among patients with preserved left ventricular (LV) ejection fraction.[14] Overall, patients with CHF and anemia tend to be older than their nonanemic counterparts.[1] The mean age of patients increased from 70.1 to 74.1 years, whereas hemoglobin concentration fell from above 13.5 to below 10.7 g/dL in a large study of 48,612 patients with a mean age of 73.2 years who were hospitalized for heart failure.[7] However, when patients with CHF are relatively young (<55 years old), the age of anemic and nonanemic patients does not appear to differ.[3]

Female Gender

The data supporting that women with CHF are at increased risk to exhibit anemia compared with

Tulane Heart and Vascular Institute, Tulane University School of Medicine, 1340 Tulane Avenue, SL-48, New Orleans, LA 70112, USA
* Corresponding author.
E-mail address: lejemtel@tulane.edu

Heart Failure Clin 6 (2010) 289–293
doi:10.1016/j.hfc.2010.03.008
1551-7136/10/$ – see front matter © 2010 Elsevier Inc. All rights reserved.

men with CHF are scarce in part because of the overwhelming proportion of men in most CHF studies. For example, a recent study of anemia in ambulatory patients with CHF reported a 64% male predominance.[15] In a population of community residents from Olmsted County that included nearly as many women as men, female gender was not found to be associated with an increased risk for developing anemia.[14] Of note, whereas the population was overwhelmingly male (77%) in their study of CHF and anemia, investigators noted that the percentage of women steadily increases from 9% to 35% as hemoglobin concentration falls from above 14.8 to below 12.3 g/dL.[3] In the previously mentioned study of patients who were found to be anemic when hospitalized for CHF deterioration, the percentage of women increased from 37.8% to 51.6% as the hemoglobin concentration fell from above 13.5 to below 10.7 g/dL.[7] Similar findings were reported in the National Heart Care project as the percentage of women rose from 43% to 61% as hematocrit fell from above 44% to below 24%.[5]

In summary, in studies of CHF and anemia that have enrolled a preponderance of men, the proportion of women steadily increases as hemoglobin concentration falls to the point that women can predominate among patients with CHF and severe anemia.

Chronic Kidney Disease

Chronic kidney disease (CKD, as defined by an estimated glomerular filtration rate [eGFR] <90 mL/min^{-1}/1.72 m^{-2}) and anemia are among the most frequent comorbid conditions in patients with CHF.[16] As expected, anemia is more prevalent in patients with CHF and CKD than in patients with CHF alone. The greater prevalence of anemia in patients with CHF and CKD compared with CHF alone has been noted in both ambulatory and hospitalized settings.[14–16] Although structural renal disease is relatively uncommon in CHF and anemia occurs in the absence of CKD, the fall in hemoglobin concentration has been repeatedly shown to closely parallel that of eGFR in large CHF registries.[7,16] The close parallel between the fall in hemoglobin concentration and eGFR provides strong albeit indirect evidence that the kidney plays a major role in the pathogenesis of anemia in CHF. For unclear reasons, patients with CHF and CKD appear to develop anemia at an eGFR than would not cause anemia in patients with only CKD. Thus, although the presence of CKD is an important determinant of low hemoglobin concentration in patients with CHF, factors other than CKD are clearly involved. In summary,

the fall in hemoglobin concentration mirrors that of eGFR in patients with CHF and the association of CHF and CKD appears to reset the eGFR threshold for developing anemia when compared with CKD alone.[17]

Functional Capacity, Hospitalization, and Fluid Retention

As expected, owing to detrimental effects of low hemoglobin concentration on oxygen delivery to peripheral tissues and nervous sympathetic and renin-angiotensin (RAS) systems activity, anemia becomes more prevalent as fatigue and shortness of breath increase in severity.[1,2] In turn, worsening symptoms tend to precipitate hospitalization and thus anemia is more frequently noted in hospitalized than in ambulatory patients. The prevalence of anemia ranges from 17.2% to 53.0% in ambulatory patients. If one uses the WHO definition of anemia, nearly three-quarters of men hospitalized for CHF decompensation present with anemia.[7,16] Hospitalization is also related to fluid retention and fluid retention commonly results in hemodilution that in turn accounts for reduced hemoglobin concentration.[18,19] When anemia is attributable to hemodilution in CHF, it carries a worse prognosis than that associated with other causes of anemia.[18] Of note, the prevalence of anemia appears to be similar in patients with CHF with reduced and preserved left ventricular (LV) ejection fraction, expansion of plasma volume is greater in patients with reduced ejection fraction than in patients with preserved ejection fraction.[20,21] Fluid retention, although not reliably detected by physical findings, is common in patients with advanced CHF.[22] In summary, as anemia exacerbates symptoms of shortness of breath and fatigue, severity of CHF and anemia are expected to be closely related. Symptomatic deterioration and fluid retention inevitably lead to hospitalization. Thus, the greater prevalence of anemia in hospitalized than ambulatory patients is expected.

SPECIFIC CAUSES OF ANEMIA
Iron Metabolism

The prevalence of iron deficiency in CHF has been reported to range from 5% to 21% in CHF. Whereas up to 73% of patients with CHF were found to have depleted bone marrow iron stores in one study, few of the patients with depleted iron stores had microcytic anemia, as their mean corpuscular volume was in the low range of normal.[23] True iron-deficiency anemia may be related to aspirin-induced occult gastrointestinal bleeding in patients with CHF. Thus, routine prescription of aspirin to patients with dilated cardiomyopathy with patent coronary arteries may result in iron-deficiency anemia. This possible adverse event of routine aspirin therapy in CHF should be kept in mind even though patients do not exhibit clear evidence of microcytic anemia. A direct link between CHF and iron-deficiency anemia has yet to be elucidated in the absence of conditions known to result in iron malabsorption such as severe right ventricular failure with gastrointestinal edema or uremic gastritis. Most investigators agree that hematinic abnormalities (iron, folate, or vitamin B12) are rare in patients with CHF.[13,24]

A commonly entertained but still unproven mechanism is that anemia in CHF resembles anemia of chronic disease as evidenced by iron acquisition by the reticuloendothelial system.[25] Plasma levels of tumor necrosis factor-α (TNF-α) and interleukin-1 and -6 (IL-1, IL-6) are elevated in severely symptomatic patients with CHF.[26] Increased levels of TNF-α and IL-6 promote storage of iron by the reticuloendothelial system and thus may result in anemia.[24] In addition, IL-6 and TNF-α inhibit renal production of erythropoietin by activating GATA 2 binding protein and nuclear factor-κB.[24] Elevated levels of TNF-α and IL-6 also tend to inhibit proliferation of bone marrow erythroid progenitor cells. Last, IL-6 may stimulate hepatic production of hepcidin that impairs duodenal iron absorption and down-regulates ferroprotein expression preventing release of iron from total body stores.[27] Anemia of chronic disease and iron-deficiency anemia may coexist in patients with CHF, and differentiating anemia of chronic disease concomitant with iron-deficiency anemia from anemia of chronic disease alone may require measurement of soluble transferrin receptors and ferritin levels to determine the ratio of transferrin receptor level over log of ferritin level.[25]

In summary, iron-deficiency anemia is relatively rare in CHF, affecting less than 10% of patients.[2] An anemia resembling that of anemia of chronic disease is far more frequently observed in patients with CHF than is iron-deficiency anemia. The precise mechanisms of this far more prevalent form of anemia are incompletely understood. Both inflammatory stress and impaired iron metabolism appear to play a role[13]; however, neither inflammatory stress nor impaired iron metabolism is unique to CHF. They may also mediate the development of anemia in chronic conditions other than CHF.[28,29]

Erythropoietin Production and Resistance

Erythropoietin, a 30.4-kDa glycoprotein growth factor, is the key component of the homeostatic system for regulation of red blood cell mass and tissue oxygen delivery.

Importantly, measurement of erythropoietin level is useful only when hemoglobin concentration falls below 10 g/dL. Above 10 g/dL, erythropoietin levels remain well above the normal range.[25] Peritubular specialized fibroblasts that are located in the cortex and outer medulla are mostly responsible for 90% of renal erythropoietin production.[2] The remaining 10% is produced by the liver. The stimulus for erythropoietin production is a fall in oxygen tension resulting in hypoxia. Renal hypoxia precipitates erythropoietin production by exponentially increasing the number of erythropoietin-producing cells.[30] Such mechanism is obviously affected by structural renal damage. In patients with CHF, renal blood flow is relatively maintained until the late stages of the syndrome, especially in patients receiving angiotensin-converting enzyme (ACE) inhibition and the renal parenchyma extracts only 10% of delivered oxygen. Thus, the fall in oxygen tension resulting in hypoxia is most likely attributable to the presence of local arteriovenous shunts in the intrarenal circulation that causes a substantial fall in oxygen tension and triggers erythropoietin production by peritubular fibroblasts. Whether highly prevalent vascular conditions such as diabetes mellitus and atherosclerosis play a role in the shunting of blood from arteriolar to venous beds remains to be studied in patients with CHF. Defective erythropoietin production was demonstrated in 92% of patients with CHF who had anemia of chronic disease as evidenced by an observed/predicted log (serum erythropoietin) ratio less than 0.8 or a defective supply for erythropoiesis diagnosed by low transferring saturation or increased soluble transferrin receptor levels.[30] In contrast to initial findings derived from a small cohort of patients with CHF (<15), erythropoietin production did not correlate with effective renal plasma flow in 97 patients with CHF.[31] The weak but significant correlation between erythropoietin production and eGFR implicates that renal dysfunction plays a role in the blunted production of erythropoietin in anemic patients.[31] Although greater than in nonanemic patients, erythropoietin levels were lower than expected for the degree of anemia, an observation that is consistent with both blunted production and resistance to erythropoietin in CHF.[30,31]

In summary, although erythropoietin levels are elevated in patients with CHF when compared with age-matched healthy subjects, the levels are below that expected for the degree of anemia. Relative bone marrow resistance to erythropoietin as observed in patients with anemia of chronic disease is also likely to contribute to lower hemoglobin concentration in CHF.

Renin-Angiotensin System

Both ACE inhibition and angiotensin receptor blockade (ARB) decrease erythropoiesis as evidenced by a decrement in hemoglobin concentration up to 0.3 g/dL. The effect of ACE inhibition and ARB lowers angiotensin II–induced decrease in local oxygen concentration that in turn triggers erythropoietin production, thereby increasing hemoglobin concentration. Angiotensin II also stimulates production of erythropoietic cells by the bone marrow.[2] Last, the amino terminal catalytic domain of ACE degrades the hematopoiesis inhibitor N-Acetyl-seryl-aspartyl-lysyl-proline (Ac-SDKP). The correlation between Ac-SDKP level and proliferation of erythroid precursor cells supports an inhibitory role of Ac-SDKP on hematopoiesis in patients with CHF, which may in part explain the fall in hemoglobin concentration in those patients receiving ACE inhibition.[32] However, experimental data in various knockout mice models involving different ACE components do not support a role for ACE inhibition in Ac-SDKP-induced degradation in reduced erythropoiesis.[33] Angiotensin II itself plays a direct role in erythropoiesis. However, its role is modest and unlikely to affect functional capacity.[34]

SUMMARY

Increased prevalence of anemia in CHF has been associated with advanced age, female gender, impaired renal function, and severity of symptoms. The underlying mechanisms of anemia in CHF largely overlap with those implicated in the anemia of chronic disease. Both impaired iron metabolism and inflammatory stress play important roles in the development and progression of anemia in CHF. The adjunct role of vascular and metabolic conditions that commonly accompany CHF has not been thoroughly investigated.

REFERENCES

1. Tang YD, Katz SD. Anemia in chronic heart failure. Prevalence, etiology, clinical correlates and treatment options. Circulation 2006;113:2454–61.
2. Anand IS. Anemia and chronic heart failure: implication and treatment options. J Am Coll Cardiol 2008;52:501–11.
3. Horwich TB, Foranow GC, Hamilton MA, et al. Anemia is associated with symptoms, greater impairment in functional capacity and a significant increase in mortality in patients with advanced heart failure. J Am Coll Cardiol 2002;39:1780–6.
4. Mozaffarian D, Nye R, Levy WC. Anemia predicts mortality in severe heart failure. The prospective randomized amlopidine survival evaluation (PRAISE). J Am Coll Cardiol 2003;41:1933–9.
5. Kosiborod M, Curtis JP, Wang Y, et al. Anemia and outcomes in patients with heart failure: a study from the National Heart Care Project. Arch Intern Med 2005;165:2237–44.
6. Groenveld HF, Januzzi JL, Damman K, et al. Anemia and mortality in heart failure. J Am Coll Cardiol 2008;52:818–27.
7. Young JB, Abraham WT, Albert NM, et al. Relation of low hemoglobin and anemia to morbidity and mortality in patients hospitalized with heart failure (insight from the OPTIMIZE-HF registry). Am J Cardiol 2008;101:223–30.
8. Izaks GJ, Westendorp RG, Knook DL. The definition of anemia in older persons. JAMA 1999;281:1714–7.
9. Ezekowitz JA, McAlister FA, Amstrong PW. Anemia is common in heart failure and is associated with poor outcomes. Circulation 2003;107:223–5.
10. Komajda M. Anemia in chronic heart failure: should we treat it and how? J Am Coll Cardiol 2007;49:763–4.
11. Clark AI, Cleland JG. Anemia and chronic heart failure. Are we asking the right questions? Circulation 2005;112:1681–3.
12. Akram K, Pearlma BL. Congestive heart failure-related anemia and a role for erythropoietin. Int J Cardiol 2007;117:296–305.
13. Allen LA, Felker GM, Mehar MR, et al. Validation and potential mechanisms of red cell distribution width as a prognostic marker of heart failure. J Card Fail 2010;16:230–8.
14. Dunlay SM, Weston SA, Redfield MM, et al. Anemia and heart failure: a community study. Am J Med 2008;121:726–32.
15. Tsang WH, Tong W, Jain A, et al. Evaluation and long-term prognosis of new-onset, transient, and persistent anemia in ambulatory patients with chronic heart failure. J Am Coll Cardiol 2008;51:569–76.
16. Go AS, Yang J, Ackerson LM, et al. Hemoglobin level, chronic kidney disease, and the risks of death and hospitalization in adults with chronic heart failure. The Anemia in Chronic Heart Failure: Outcomes and Resources Utilization (ANCHOR) study. Circulation 2006;113:2713–23.
17. Luthi JC, Flanders WD, Burnier M, et al. Anemia of chronic and kidney disease are associated with poor outcomes in heart failure patients. BMC Nephrol 2006;7:3.
18. Androne AS, Katz SD, Lund L, et al. Hemodilution is common in patients with advanced heart failure. Circulation 2003;107:226–9.
19. Mancini DM, Katz SD, Lang CC, et al. Effect of anemia on exercise capacity in patients with

moderate to severe chronic heart failure. Circulation 2003;107:294–9.

20. Abramov D, Cohen RS, Katz SD, et al. Comparison of blood volume characteristics in anemia patients with low versus preserved left ventricular ejection fractions. Am J Cardiol 2008;102:1069–73.

21. Brucks S, Little WC, Chao T, et al. Relation of anemia to diastolic heart failure and the effect on outcome. Am J Cardiol 2004;93:1055–7.

22. Androne AS, Hryniewicz K, Hudaihed A. Relation of unrecognized hypervolemia in chronic heart failure to clinical status, hemodynamic and patient outcomes. Am J Cardiol 2004;93:1254–9.

23. Nanas JN, Matsouka C, Karageorgopoulos D, et al. Etiology of anemia in patients with advanced heart failure. J Am Coll Cardiol 2006;48:2485–9.

24. Dec WC. Anemia and iron deficiency—new therapeutic targets in heart failure? N Engl J Med 2009;361:2475–7.

25. Weiss G, Goodnough LT. Anemia of chronic disease. N Engl J Med 2005;352:1011–23.

26. Testa M, Yeh M, Fanelli R, et al. Circulating levels of cytokines and their endogenous modulators in patients with mild to severe congestive heart failure due to coronary artery disease and hypertension. J Am Coll Cardiol 1996;28:964–71.

27. Ganz T. Hepcidin: a key regulator of iron metabolism and mediator of anemia of inflammation. Blood 2003;102:783–8.

28. John M, Lange A, Hoenig S, et al. Prevalence of anemia in chronic obstructive pulmonary disease: comparison to other chronic diseases. Int J Cardiol 2006;111:365–70.

29. Chatila WM, Thomashow BM, Minai OA, et al. Comorbidities in chronic obstructive pulmonary disease. Proc Am Thorac Soc 2008;5:549–55.

30. Opasich C, Cazzola M, Scelsi L, et al. Blunted erythropoietin production and defective iron supply for erythropoiesis as major causes of anaemia in patients with chronic heart failure. Eur Heart J 2005;26:2232–7.

31. Westenbrink BD, Visser FW, Voors AA, et al. Anaemia in chronic heart failure is not only related to impaired renal perfusion and blunted erythropoietin production but to fluid retention as well. Eur Heart J 2007;28:166–71.

32. van der Meer P, Lipsic E, Westrenbrink BD, et al. Levels of hematopoiesis inhibitor N-acetyl-seryl-aspartyl-lysyl–proline partially explain the occurrence of anemia in heart failure. Circulation 2005;112:1743–7.

33. Bernstein KE, Xiao HD, Frenzel K, et al. Six truisms concerning ACE and the renin-angiotensin system educed from the genetic analysis of mice. Circ Res 2005;96:1135–44.

34. Ghali JK, Anand IS, Abraham WT, et al. Randomized double-blind trial of darbepoietin alfa in patients with symptomatic heart failure. Circulation 2008;117:526–35.

Molecular Changes in Myocardium in the Course of Anemia or Iron Deficiency

Ewa A. Jankowska, MD, PhD, FESC*,
Piotr Ponikowski, MD, PhD, FESC

KEYWORDS

• Myocardium • Anemia • Iron deficiency • Hemodynamics

The links between anemia, iron deficiency (ID) and impaired hemodynamics were suggested more than 50 years ago, but remained neglected.[1,2] Chronic untreated anemia or ID can result in an increased cardiac output, chronic sympathetic activation, left ventricular hypertrophy, and left ventricular dilation, leading to symptomatic chronic heart failure (CHF). Only in the past decade have clinicians and scientists gained interest In anemia and ID occurring in the course of CHF.

Anemia constitutes an important comorbidity in patients with CHF, with a prevalence ranging from 10% to 55%, depending on the severity of heart disease in examined patients and the applied criteria for the diagnosis of anemia.[3,4] The presence of anemia has crucial clinical and prognostic consequences in patients with CHF, because it is related to impaired exercise capacity, poor quality of life, high hospitalization rates, and fatal outcome.[3–7]

The pathogenesis of anemia occurring in the course of CHF is complex, and has not yet been comprehensively established.[3,8,9] The following elements are likely to be involved in the development of anemia in patients with CHF: renal failure, inflammation, reduced erythropoietin (EPO) production and EPO resistance, absolute and functional ID, diabetes, hemodilution, gastrointestinal blood loss, and therapy with angiotensin-converting enzyme inhibitors and/or angiotensin receptor blockers.[3,8,9]

Anemia found in patients with CHF represents an anemia of chronic diseases (ACD), being of an immunologic origin.[10] CHF is a state characterized by an augmented generalized inflammation with high circulating levels of proinflammatory cytokines (interleukin-1 [IL-1], interleukin-6 [IL-6], tumor necrosis factor α [TNF-α]).[8,10] These molecules are directly involved in the development of 2 pathologies playing a central role in the pathophysiology of anemia in CHF, namely EPO resistance (an impaired responsiveness of target hematopoietic and extrahematopoietic cells to EPO) and functional ID (iron stores trapped inside the cells of the reticuloendothelial system).[9–11] In the context of CHF, interest in ID is increasing not only as a causal factor leading to or aggravating anemia but also as a separate pathology (without concomitant anemia) with serious unfavorable consequences for the general homeostasis of an organism, including survival.[12,13]

Patients with CHF and concomitant anemia or ID develop structural and molecular changes within the cardiovascular system and most peripheral tissues and organs. Some changes occurring in patients with CHF with concomitant anemia or ID are the direct consequences of these pathologies. However, the multifactorial origin of anemia

Department of Heart Diseases, Wroclaw Medical University, Centre for Heart Diseases, Military Hospital, ul Weigla 5, Wroclaw 50-981, Poland
* Corresponding author.
E-mail address: ewa@antro.pan.wroc.pl

Heart Failure Clin 6 (2010) 295–304
doi:10.1016/j.hfc.2010.03.003
1551-7136/10/$ – see front matter © 2010 Elsevier Inc. All rights reserved.

or ID in CHF makes elucidating the effects of these pathologies on cardiovascular and other target tissues is a difficult task because the other derangements accompanying anemia or ID (such as renal dysfunction and inflammation) may markedly interfere with the studied pathomechanisms and relationships.

This article discusses the consequences of impaired EPO signaling and deranged iron metabolism on the functioning and structure of myocardium in experimental and clinical models. Derangements within EPO signaling and iron metabolism occurring in CHF and other clinical settings affect the functioning and structure of most body tissues and organs (eg, skeletal muscles, central nervous system, immune competent cells, and kidneys).[14–16] These effects are particularly important in the context of CHF because virtually all body tissues and organs are affected, but these issues are beyond the scope of this article.

ROLE OF EPO IN CHF

As mentioned earlier, in CHF high circulating levels of proinflammatory cytokines disrupt the EPO metabolism and subsequently the effectiveness of erythropoiesis in at least 2 ways.[9,10] They inhibit the renal production of EPO (the reduced EPO secretion in response to the hypoxic stimulus) and induce the EPO resistance (within hematopoietic and extrahematopoietic cells).[9,10] In the study by Opasich and colleagues,[17] 57% of 148 patients with anemia with CHF had an ACD, and 92% showed reduced production of endogenous EPO. Other mechanisms that could explain EPO resistance occurring in CHF include ID, blood loss, infections, malignancy, secondary hyperparathyroidism, vitamin B_{12} or folate deficiencies, intrinsic bone marrow dysfunction, red cell enzyme defects, hemolysis, and interactions with certain drugs.[3,9]

Patients with CHF have increased serum levels of EPO in proportion to the severity of heart disease.[18,19] In this group of patients (and in contrast to healthy subjects), there is only a weak inverse association between circulating EPO and hemoglobin level, which may suggest a blunted EPO response relative to hemoglobin levels and even a resistance to EPO within bone marrow.[18] CHF may impair the functioning of bone marrow. It has been shown that an induction of CHF in mice is followed by a reduction in the bone marrow proerythroblast population, with impaired proliferative capacity and augmented apoptosis of these cells.[20] However, the upregulated expression of EPO receptor in failing hearts in mice may suggest

the presence of EPO resistance or relative EPO deficiency in target tissues.[21] High EPO levels predict unfavorable outcomes in patients with CHF, independently of hemoglobin levels and other clinically established prognosticators.[18,19] More importantly, patients with anemia and CHF who have EPO levels higher than expected (suggesting the presence of EPO resistance) have a significantly higher mortality than those with EPO levels equal to or lower than expected, also after adjustment for standard prognosticators including age, hemoglobin level, plasma N-terminal pro–brain natriuretic peptide (NT-proBNP), and renal function.[22]

CARDIOPROTECTIVE EPO SIGNALING

EPO (also a hematopoietic cytokine) is no longer considered only as a regulator of hematopoiesis.[9,23–28] EPO is a hormone involved in the regulation of proliferation and differentiation of erythroid cells, but EPO also has several pleiotropic effects on diverse nonhematopoietic target tissues.[9,26–28] EPO is synthesized not only by kidneys but also locally by many extrarenal tissues (eg, bone marrow, brain, liver, spleen, reproductive organs), especially in conditions of metabolic or oxidative stress, or any other injury.[23–25] All tissues producing EPO (and some others) express the specific EPO receptors and are able to respond to this hormone.[23–25]

There is increasing evidence that myocardium is also a target for EPO.[9,27,28] The presence of EPO receptors within the adult rat heart tissue on endothelial cells, fibroblasts and differentiated cardiomyocytes,[29] human and bovine endothelial cells,[30] human vascular smooth muscle cells,[31] human atrial and ventricular cardiomyocytes,[32] and murine and rabbit cardiofibroblasts [33–35] suggests that these cells are responsive to EPO stimulation. EPO signaling for heart homoeostasis seems to be of crucial importance, because mice deficient in genes for EPO or EPO receptor develop severe ventricular hypoplasia with a reduced number of proliferative cardiomyocytes and significant pathologies within cardiac vasculature.[36] EPO reveals no protective effects on adult cardiomyocytes in mice lacking EPO receptor in an experimental model of staurosporine-induced apoptosis.[37]

There is no consensus on whether EPO can be synthesized within normal or failing myocardium. Some investigators have failed to confirm the expression of EPO in the heart under normoxic or mild hypoxic conditions.[38] Hypoxic cardiomyocytes can produce hypoxia inducible factor 1α (HIF-1α),[39] which is critical for the upregulation of

EPO transcription in all cells. This observation has led to the hypothesis that myocardium might produce EPO locally. Some investigators have shown the presence of EPO within rat myocardium, based on immunostaining.[40] Only recently has the transcription of EPO mRNA and the presence of EPO protein been confirmed within porcine myocardium exposed to pyruvate-fortified cardioplegia during postsurgical recovery after cardiopulmonary bypass.[41] In this model, the increase in EPO expression was accompanied by the augmented cardioprotective EPO signaling mechanisms in porcine myocardium.[41] These experimental findings need to be reassessed in clinical settings.

EPO has an analogous molecular structure and acts via a similar intracellular signaling pathways as the family of type 1 cytokines.[23,26,42–44] Interacting with its specific receptors (which belong to the cytokine receptor superfamily), EPO activates several transcriptional factors, and, as a result, generally suppresses apoptosis and promotes survival and growth in various cell types.[23,26,42–44] The intracellular mechanisms of EPO are not fully understood. EPO mediates cardioprotection by multiple intracellular signaling pathways that are not redundant.[26,45] The interaction of EPO with its specific receptors results in the dimerization of EPO receptor and the induction of several intracellular signaling cascades also within cardiomyocytes,[23,24,26–28,42,46] namely: (1) the activation of janus tyrosine kinase (JAK)/signal transducer and activator of transcription (STAT) pathway (the promotion of survival signaling in cardiomyocytes[47]); (2) the activation of phosphatidylinositol 3-kinase (PI3 K)/serine threonine protein kinase B (Akt) pathway (the reduction in myocardial apoptosis and caspase-3 activation by ischemia/reperfusion injury in the isolated perfused rat heart,[48] the inhibition of glycogen synthase kinase 3b, and subsequently the reduction of mitochondrial injury, lower leakage of cytochrome c, and inhibited apoptosis[49]); (3) the activation of phospholipase C (PCK)/protein kinase C pathway (the activation of sarcolemmal and mitochondrial K^+ ATP channels and membrane voltage-sensitive Ca^{2+} channel in cardiomyocytes[50]); (4) the activation of RAS/mitogen-activated protein kinase (MAPK) pathway (the promotion of cellular survival, growth, and differentiation[45]); (5) the inhibition of nuclear factor κB (NF-κB) and activator protein 1 (AP-1) pathway (the attenuation of the proinflammatory cytokines TNF-α and IL-6, and the enhancement of the anti-inflammatory cytokine IL-10[51]).

Some effects of EPO result from enhanced nitric oxide (NO) bioavailability through an induction of endothelial NO synthase (eNOS) transcription and an activation of this enzyme.[52,53] NO poses several advantageous properties: for example, it is a strong vasodilator and modulator of vascular tone[54,55]; and an inhibitor of platelet adhesion and aggregation,[56,57] smooth muscle cell migration,[58] and leukocyte adhesion.[59] Transgenic mice with an overexpression of EPO are characterized by an increased eNOS expression, higher NO release, and greater NO-mediated vascular relaxation, which prevents them from developing myocardial infarction and heart dysfunction compared with wild type animals.[60] EPO can induce eNOS expression in bone marrow, which is crucial for the recruitment and mobilization of endothelial progenitor cells (EPCs).[53]

CHANGES IN MYOCARDIUM DUE TO IMPROVED EPO SIGNALING

Currently, pleiotropic effects of EPO are of particular interest, in particular in the context of potential novel therapeutic approaches for patients with CHF that may arise from specific cellular mechanisms of EPO.[9,27,28] In general, EPO plays a protective-restorative role in various tissues through an activation of cytoprotection, a reduction of inflammatory responses, an increase in vascular integrity, a mobilization of stem cells, an induction of proliferation and differentiation, a promotion of cell survival, and an inhibition of cell apoptosis.[23–25]

Analogous EPO properties have been found regarding myocardium.[9,27,28] There is increasing evidence of the protective role of EPO in experimental models of myocardial infarction and ischemia/reperfusion injury, during the acute phase of injury and during the longer period after the heart damage, which lead to attenuated cardiac remodeling.[29,33,34,61–63]

According to Parsa and colleagues,[34,62] an administration of EPO reveals antiapoptotic effects in vitro on embryonic rat myoblasts and in vivo on rabbit cardiomyocytes exposed to ischemic/reperfusion injury or experimental myocardial infarction. In the study by Calvillo and colleagues,[63] EPO therapy prevents the apoptosis of cultured adult rat cardiomyocytes exposed to hypoxia. In isolated rat hearts, perfusion with EPO during ischemia/reperfusion injury reduces cellular damage, diminishes apoptosis, and improves the recovery of left ventricular pressure and blood flow compared with nonperfused organs.[29] EPO-treated rabbits and rats show a smaller infarct size, reduced apoptosis within the infarcted area, and improved inotropic reserve compared with untreated animals.[34,62] Mutant mice that expressed EPO receptors only on hematopoietic cells showed increased caspase-3 activity and more terminal deoxynucleotide transferase-mediated dUTP nick-end labeling (TUNEL)-positive (apoptotic) cardiomyocytes within the ischemic area in the experimental model of ischemia/reperfusion injury compared with wild type rodents.[64]

EPO signaling is also involved in the recruitment and activation of circulating bone marrow–derived EPCs and CD34+, which participate in the regenerative processes within the cardiovascular system, being responsible for endothelial and vascular repair in patients with renal failure, CHF, and healthy subjects.[65–67] In patients with renal anemia, a treatment with EPO increases the number of all circulating EPCs and functionally active EPCs.[67,68] The stimulatory effects on EPCs can be observed even at subtherapeutic EPO doses with respect to the correction of renal anemia.[67] Activating some prosurvival cellular pathways, EPO makes EPCs more resistant to ischemic stimuli.[69] In an experimental rat model, EPO has been shown to improve cardiac function even when started 3 weeks after ischemia/reperfusion injury, and the beneficial effects were related mainly to an increased number of circulating EPCs.[29] In rats with doxorubicin-induced cardiomyopathy EPO, administration activated the mobilization of EPCs.[70]

There is also evidence that, in neonatal rat cardiomyocytes, EPO can increase the NA^+/K^+ATP-ase activity,[71] mobilize intracellular Ca^{2+},[42,72] and induce a broad range of other cellular responses, including mitogenesis, chemotaxis, and angiogenesis in various peripheral tissues (including skeletal and myocardial muscles).[24,42]

Several investigators have shown antiinflammatory properties of EPO in the context of the cardiovascular system. In in vitro models, EPO antagonizes the effects of proinflammatory cytokines (such as IL-6, TNF-α, monocyte chemotactic protein 1 [MCP-1])[73] and protects against lipopolysaccharide-mediated apoptosis.[74] Administration of EPO results in a reduction of levels of inflammatory markers and cytokines in experimental models of myocardial infarction.[51] EPO therapy started 6 weeks after an induction of a large myocardial infarction in mice resulted in diminished left ventricular dilatation, improved cardiac function, reduction of inflammatory cell infiltration and fibrosis in the myocardium, and near normalization of the high levels of proinflammatory cytokines seen in failing hearts.[21]

Studies in patients with chronic renal failure have found that EPO therapy can reduce exercise-induced myocardial ischemia in subjects with coronary artery diseases.[75] EPO administration can also ameliorate left ventricular hypertrophy.[63,76] In anemic patients with CHF (with and without chronic renal failure), a correction of anemia with EPO and oral iron after 1 year improves left and right ventricular systolic function and reduces circulating BNP levels.[77,78]

In a view of the multiple cellular effects of EPO, it is presumed that therapy with EPO in subjects with CHF is beyond modifying hematopoiesis itself and reversing anemia, but other cellular phenomena occurring on the level of failing myocardium are of major clinical significance. Beneficial effects of EPO therapy in subjects with CHF can result from the modulation of erythropoiesis and from the direct interaction with the myocardium, and it is difficult to distinguish between these mechanisms in experimental and clinical models.

There are few lines of evidence suggesting that the cardiovascular effects of EPO in subjects with CHF are, at least to some extent, due to the direct interaction of EPO with myocardial EPO receptors. First, cultured cardiomyocytes and isolated perfused hearts can respond to the direct exposition to EPO in in vitro models.[63,79] Second, the reactions within the cardiovascular system as a consequence of EPO administration are observed earlier (after the single dose) before the changes that occur within the erythroid system.[62] Third, it has been shown that low-dose EPO therapy administered for 9 weeks in rats with ischemic CHF had no effect on hematocrit, but such an intervention improved cardiac function, induced neovascularization, and attenuated a switch to slow β myosin heavy chain (MHC) isoforms.[80] Fourth, modified EPO (carbamylated EPO [CEPO]), with no affinity to EPO receptors, and hence lacking the effects on erythropoiesis, revealed its cardioprotective properties in experimental models of chronic ischemia[81] and ischemia/reperfusion injury.[82]

ROLE OF ID IN CHF

Iron plays a crucial role in oxygen transport (as a component of hemoglobin), oxygen storage (as a component of myoglobin), and oxidative metabolism in the skeletal and heart muscle (as a component of oxidative enzymes and respiratory chain proteins).[83,84] The maintenance of normal iron metabolism is critical for tissues that have high mitogenic potential (neoplastic cells, hematopoietic cells, immune competent cells) and high energy demand (hepatocytes, adipocytes, renal cells, immune cells, skeletal myocytes, cardiomyocytes).[85–90] The presence of ID has numerous clinical consequences that are directly related not only to impaired erythropoiesis but also to marked impairment of oxidative metabolism, cellular energetics, and cellular immune mechanisms.[83–91] ID with and without anemia is accompanied by reduced aerobic capacity,[92] and its correction improves symptomatic performance and exercise tolerance in patients with CHF.[93,94]

Evidence on the epidemiology and pathophysiology of ID in CHF is scarce, and there is no gold standard to diagnose ID in CHF. ID has usually only been considered in the context of anemia, in a general population and in patients with CHF. In the study by Ezekowitz and colleagues,[95] anemia was present in 17% of incident hospital discharges for heart failure, and ID was the confirmed cause of anemia in 21%. Opasich and colleagues[17] found that, among 148 anemic patients with CHF, 57% had an ACD, and in this group nearly all (92%) had defective iron supply for erythropoiesis or blunted endogenous EPO production. Nanas and colleagues[96] investigated hospitalized patients with anemia and advanced CHF (all New York Heart Association [NYHA] class IV) and, based on bone marrow biopsies, showed that 73% presented with ID.

Patients with CHF are prone to become iron deficient secondarily to a depletion of iron stores (absolute ID) or, more frequently, as a result of impaired iron metabolism in the course of generalized inflammation occurring in CHF (functional ID).[10,11,97] Also in the course of CHF, proinflammatory cytokines block intestinal absorption of iron and divert iron from the circulation into the reticuloendothelial system, causing reticuloendothelial block.[97] Hepcidin, a small hepatic peptide, secreted in response to proinflammatory cytokines, seems to play a key role in the control of these processes.[98,99] Decreased intestinal iron absorption, together with its accumulation within the reticuloendothelial stores, reduces iron availability to its target tissues and organs.[98,99] Therefore, functional ID may occur despite adequate iron stores in the body, in contrast to absolute ID, when the iron stores are significantly depleted.

The pattern of changes in circulating levels of hepcidin in the course of CHF remains unclear. In a small pilot study by Suzuki and colleagues,[100] patients during the acute phase of myocardial infarction showed increased serum levels of hepcidin-20 and hepcidin-25. In these patients, there were no associations between circulating hepcidin and markers of inflammation (IL-6, C-reactive protein); however, a small number of examined patients requires a cautious interpretation.[100] In another pilot study, by Matsumoto and colleagues,[101] patients with anemia and CHF had reduced serum hepcidin-25 levels compared with controls and patients without anemia with CHF. In this study, anemic subjects did not show increased IL-6 levels. Among patients with anemia and CHF, circulating hepcidin correlated positively with serum ferritin (suggesting links with depleted body iron storage), and negatively with serum EPO (EPO is known to suppress the hepatic synthesis of hepcidin). There was no relationship between circulating hepcidin-25 and IL-6 in the examined group of patients.[101] In this study, patients with anemia and CHF probably showed mainly absolute ID (without an activation of inflammatory processes) with low ferritin level accompanied by reduced hepcidin.

The authors have applied a definition of ID taking into account absolute (serum ferritin <100 µg/dL) and functional ID (serum ferritin ≥100 µg/dL and <300 µg/dL when transferin saturation [Tsat] <20%).[13,93] We have shown that the prevalence of ID was 37% in the entire group of 546 patients with systolic CHF (32% vs 57% in subjects without vs with anemia defined as hemoglobin level <12 g/dL in women and <13 g/dL in men, $P<.001$).[13] The presence of ID, as defined earlier, was a strong and independent predictor of poor outcome in patients with CHF, irrespective of clinical status and the concurrence of anemia.[13]

CHANGES IN MYOCARDIUM DUE TO ID

Iron constitutes an important element of the enzymatic system of cardiomyocytes, and can be stored inside these cells. Molecular elements of the iron metabolism system are present within healthy, failing, and inflamed myocardium.[102–105] However, available evidence on their role in the physiology and pathophysiology of myocardium remains scarce.

Turner and colleagues[106] have shown that rats with induced ID show increased cardiac output and sympathetic activation that subsequently result in left ventricular hypertrophy, an increased abdominal aorta diameter (suggesting the flow-dependent remodeling of the arterial wall), and an increased distensibility (suggesting the reduction in arterial collagen content). Links between ID and the development of left ventricular hypertrophy have been confirmed by several investigators in experimental models.[107–112] Iron is necessary for collagen synthesis, and the quantity of collagen is reduced in myocardium from iron-deficient animals.[113] Dong and colleagues[112] reported that left ventricular hypertrophy and dilatation occurring in iron-deficient rats is accompanied by mitochondrial swelling and irregular sarcomere organization, increased mitochondrial cytochrome c release, and increased reactive nitrogen species expression in cardiomyocytes, suggesting the critical role of normal iron metabolism for energetics and oxidative balance in exercising tissues (such as myocardium).

The iron-regulatory hormone hepcidin has been found in myocardium from healthy rats.[102] The expression of iron exporters required for iron release from mammalian cells (ferroportin, ceruloplasmin, hephaestin)[103,104] has also been found in hearts from rats and in cardiomyocyte cultures. Hepcidin is also present in cardiomyocytes from rats with experimental autoimmune myocarditis and acute myocardial infarction, and in human hearts with myocarditis.[105]

The role of proteins regulating iron metabolism within cardiomyocytes remains unclear. Ge and colleagues[103] established that hepcidin is able to bind with, internalize, and degrade ferroportin (its membrane receptor), and then decrease iron export in H9C2 cardiomyocytes (a permanent cell line derived from the embryonic rat ventricle), leading to an abnormal increase in heart iron and iron-mediated cell injury.[103] These investigators also showed that hepcidin did not interact with ceruloplasmin or hephaestin.[103]

Isoda and colleagues[105] found positive correlations between the expression of hepcidin and IL-6, as well as between the expression of BNP and IL-6, within cardiomyocytes from ischemic and inflamed myocardium, suggesting links between deranged iron metabolism and inflammation present locally within myocardium. In vivo hypoxia and an induction of acute-phase inflammation can lead to a strong upregulation of hepcidin expression on mRNA and protein levels in the heart, with the accompanying increased immunoreactivity of hepcidin at the myocardial intercalated disc area.[102] It is presumed that hepcidin synthesized locally in the heart may be involved in cardiac pathologies.[102]

Naito andcolleagues[114] investigated the molecular mechanisms of the adaptive and maladaptive responses of myocardium to 20-week anemia induced by ID in male rats. After 12 weeks, ID anemia resulted in compensated cardiac hypertrophy with preserved cardiac output. At this time, circulating EPO levels and the phosphorylation of signal transducer and activation of transcription 3 (STAT3) in myocardium increased, and revealed favorable effects on the structure and function of myocardium.[114] After 20 weeks, iron-deficient anemic rats developed maladapted cardiac hypertrophy with severe left ventricular dysfunction, and presented signs of decompensation (lung congestion). Dilated ventricles were characterized by myocardial interstitial fibrosis and an increased myocardial expression of

A-type natriuretic peptide (ANP) and BNP, and as well as a reduced myocardial expression of collagen type 3 genes.[114] At this point, a significant decrease in serum EPO, an increase in EPO receptor expression on cardiomyocytes, and a concomitant reduction in phosphorylated STAT3 within failing myocardium occurred; all these changes revealed detrimental effects on myocardium.[114] The administration of EPO in a subgroup of animals at the stage of compensated cardiac hypertrophy prevented the development of heart dysfunction, suggesting the role of EPO and iron in integrative heart functioning.[114]

Toblli and colleagues[40] assessed the effect of an induction of renal failure, anemia with accompanying ID in rats on left ventricular function, and structure. Male rats underwent subtotal nephrectomy that, after 6 months, resulted in a marked reduction in creatinine clearance, hemoglobin level, serum iron, and transferrin saturation, and an increase in arterial blood pressure compared with sham-operated animals.[40] The corresponding surgery induced the development of left ventricular hypertrophy and a reduction of fraction of shortening (FS), and a low FS was accompanied by reduced hemoglobin and hypoferremia, suggesting an involvement of anemia and ID in the pathogenesis of heart dysfunction.[40]

Prussian blue staining showed a significant amount of iron in hypertrophied hearts, but serum and tissue ferritin levels were decreased, suggesting the presence of functional ID. Cardiomyocytes from hypertrophied hearts showed an increased expression of proinflammatory cytokines (IL-6, TNF-α), markers of apoptosis (caspase-3), HIF-1α, EPO, and hepcidin, compared with tissues from sham-operated animals.[40] This is the first evidence suggesting that anemia and ID present in peripheral blood is accompanied by analogous changes within target extrahematopoietic tissues, such as myocardium. The cardiomyocytes from animals with subtotal nephrectomy showed features of inflammation, hypoxia, and a local upregulation of EPO transcription.[40] All these factors may lead to the augmented expression of hepcidin and the induction of functional ID, seen also on the tissue level. There were negative correlations between semiquantitative staining for hepcidin and FS%, and between serum iron and semiquantitative staining for caspase-3, suggesting the involvement of deranged iron metabolism in cardiomyocyte apoptosis, myocardial remodeling, and heart dysfunction.[40]

The study by Toblli and colleagues[40] suggests that an anemia induced by ID results in the development of functional ID within myocardium with unfavorable changes regarding its structure and function. These experimental data need to be confirmed in clinical settings in patients with renal failure and/or CHF.

SUMMARY

The pharmacologic support in EPO signaling or the correction in iron metabolism may activate molecular pathways that can protect the heart and prevent myocardial remodeling, and hence become a novel therapeutic approach in patients with CHF. Most of the data come from experimental models. Further studies, in particular performed in clinical settings, are warranted.

REFERENCES

1. Somers K. Acute reversible heart failure in severe iron-deficiency anemia associated with hookworm infestation in Uganda Africans. Circulation 1959; 19:672–5.
2. Duke M, Abelmann WH. The hemodynamic response to chronic anemia. Circulation 1969;39: 503–15.
3. Silverberg DS, Wexler D, Iaina A, et al. The role of correction of anemia in patients with congestive heart failure: a short review. Eur J Heart Fail 2008; 10:819–23.
4. Tang YD, Katz SD. The prevalence of anemia in chronic heart failure and its impact on the clinical outcomes. Heart Fail Rev 2008;13:387–92.
5. Anand IS, Kuskowski MA, Rector TS, et al. Anemia and change in hemoglobin over time related to mortality and morbidity in patients with chronic heart failure: results from Val-HeFT. Circulation 2005;112:1121–7.
6. Komajda M, Anker SD, Charlesworth A, et al. The impact of new onset anemia on morbidity and mortality in chronic heart failure: results from COMET. Eur Heart J 2006;27:1440–6.
7. Tang WH, Tong W, Jain A, et al. Evaluation and long-term prognosis of new-onset, transient, and persistent anemia in ambulatory patients with chronic heart failure. J Am Coll Cardiol 2008;51: 569–76.
8. Anand IS. Heart failure and anemia: mechanisms and pathophysiology. Heart Fail Rev 2008;13: 379–86.
9. Manolis AS, Tzeis S, Triantafyllou K, et al. Erythropoietin in heart failure and other cardiovascular diseases: hematopoietic and pleiotropic effects. Curr Drug Targets Cardiovasc Haematol Disord 2005;5:355–75.
10. Weiss G. Iron metabolism in the anemia of chronic disease. Biochim Biophys Acta 2009;1790:682–93.
11. Balla J, Jeney V, Varga Z, et al. Iron homeostasis in chronic inflammation. Acta Physiol Hung 2007;94: 95–106.
12. Anker SD, Colet JC, Filippatos G, et al. FAIR-HF committees and investigators. Rationale and design of Ferinject Assessment in patients with IRon deficiency and chronic Heart Failure (FAIR-HF) study: a randomized, placebo-controlled study of intravenous iron supplementation in patients with and without anemia. Eur J Heart Fail 2009;11:1084–91.
13. Jankowska EA, Rozentryt P, Witkowska A, et al. Iron deficiency: an ominous sign in patients with systolic chronic heart failure. Eur Heart J 2010, in press.
14. Brines ML, Ghezzi P, Keenan S, et al. Erythropoietin crosses the blood-brain barrier to protect against experimental brain injury. Proc Natl Acad Sci U S A 2000;97:10526–31.
15. Scoppetta C, Grassi F. Erythropoietin: a new tool for muscle disorders? Med Hypotheses 2004;63: 73–5.
16. Noguchi CT, Wang L, Rogers HM, et al. Survival and proliferative roles of erythropoietin beyond the erythroid lineage. Expert Rev Mol Med 2008; 10:e36.
17. Opasich C, Cazzola M, Scelsi L, et al. Blunted erythropoietin production and defective iron supply for erythropoiesis as major causes of anemia in patients with chronic heart failure. Eur Heart J 2005;26:2232–7.
18. van der Moor P, Voors AA, Lipsic E, et al. Prognostic value of plasma erythropoietin on mortality in patients with chronic heart failure. J Am Coll Cardiol 2004;44:63–7.
19. George J, Patal S, Wexler D, et al. Circulating erythropoietin levels and prognosis in patients with congestive heart failure: comparison with neurohormonal and inflammatory markers. Arch Intern Med 2005;165:1304–9.
20. Iversen PO, Woldbaek PR, Tønnessen T, et al. Decreased hematopoiesis in bone marrow of mice with congestive heart failure. Am J Physiol Regul Integr Comp Physiol 2002;282:R166–72.
21. Li Y, Takemura G, Okada H, et al. Reduction of inflammatory cytokine expression and oxidative damage by erythropoietin in chronic heart failure. Cardiovasc Res 2006;71:684–94.
22. van der Meer P, Lok DJ, Januzzi JL, et al. Adequacy of endogenous erythropoietin levels and mortality in anaemic heart failure patients. Eur Heart J 2008;29:1510–5.
23. Maiese K, Li F, Chong ZZ. New avenues of exploration for erythropoietin. JAMA 2005; 293:90–5.
24. Lappin TR, Maxwell AP, Johnston PG. EPO's alter ego: erythropoietin has multiple actions. Stem Cells 2002;20:485–92.

25. Jelkmann W, Wagner K. Beneficial and ominous aspects of the pleiotropic action of erythropoietin. Ann Hematol 2004;83:673–86.

26. Foley RN. Erythropoietin: physiology and molecular mechanisms. Heart Fail Rev 2008;13:405–14.

27. Latini R, Brines M, Fiordaliso F. Do non-hemopoietic effects of erythropoietin play a beneficial role in heart failure? Heart Fail Rev 2008;13:415–23.

28. Marzo F, Lavorgna A, Coluzzi G, et al. Erythropoietin in heart and vessels: focus on transcription and signalling pathways. J Thromb Thrombolysis 2008;26:183–7.

29. van der Meer P, Lipsic E, Henning RH, et al. Erythropoietin improves left ventricular function and coronary flow in an experimental model of ischemia-reperfusion injury. Eur J Heart Fail 2004;6:853–9.

30. Anagnostou A, Liu Z, Steiner M, et al. Erythropoietin receptor mRNA expression in human endothelial cells. Proc Natl Acad Sci U S A 1994;91:3974–8.

31. Brines M, Cerami A. Discovering erythropoietin's extrahematopoietic functions: biology and clinical promise. Kidney Int 2006;70:246–50.

32. Depping R, Kawakami K, Ocker H, et al. Expression of the erythropoietin receptor in human heart. J Thorac Cardiovasc Surg 2005;130:877–8.

33. Lipsic E, Schoemaker RG, van der Meer P, et al. Protective effects of erythropoietin in cardiac ischemia. J Am Coll Cardiol 2006;48:2161–7.

34. Parsa CJ, Kim J, Riel RU, et al. Cardioprotective effects of erythropoietin in the reperfused ischemic heart: a potential role for cardiac fibroblasts. J Biol Chem 2004;279:20655–62.

35. van der Meer P, Voors AA, Lipsic E, et al. Erythropoietin in cardiovascular diseases. Eur Heart J 2004;25:285–91.

36. Wu H, Lee SH, Gao J, et al. Inactivation of erythropoietin leads to defects in cardiac morphogenesis. Development 1999;126:3597–605.

37. Brines M, Grasso G, Fiordaliso F, et al. Erythropoietin mediates tissue protection through an erythropoietin and common beta-subunit heteroreceptor. Proc Natl Acad Sci U S A 2004;101:14907–12.

38. Heidbreder M, Frohlich F, Johren O, et al. Hypoxia rapidly activates HIF-3alpha mRNA expression. FASEB J 2003;17:1541–3.

39. Jung F, Palmer LA, Zhou N, et al. Hypoxic regulation of inducible nitric oxide synthase via hypoxia inducible factor-1 in cardiac myocytes. Circ Res 2000;86:319–25.

40. Toblli JE, Cao G, Rivas C, et al. Heart and iron deficiency anemia in rats with renal insufficiency: the role of hepcidin. Nephrology (Carlton) 2008;13:636–45.

41. Ryou MG, Flaherty DC, Hoxha B, et al. Pyruvate-fortified cardioplegia evokes myocardial erythropoietin signaling in swine undergoing cardiopulmonary bypass. Am J Physiol Heart Circ Physiol 2009;297:H1914–1922.

42. Smith KJ, Bleyer AJ, Little WC, et al. The cardiovascular effects of erythropoietin. Cardiovasc Res 2003;59:538–48.

43. Ozaki K, Leonard WJ. Cytokine and cytokine receptor pleiotropy and redundancy. J Biol Chem 2002;277:29355–8.

44. D'Andrea AD, Zon L. Erythropoietin receptor. Subunit, structure and activation. J Clin Invest 1990;86:681–7.

45. Baker JE. Erythropoietin mimics ischemic preconditioning. Vascul Pharmacol 2005;42:233–41.

46. Farrell F, Lee A. The erythropoietin receptor and its expression in tumor cells and other tissues. Oncologist 2004;9(Suppl 5):18–30.

47. Rafiee P, Shi Y, Su J, et al. Erythropoietin protects the infant heart against ischemia-reperfusion injury by triggering multiple signaling pathways. Basic Res Cardiol 2005;100:187–97.

48. Cai Z, Semenza GL. Phosphatidylinositol-3-kinase signaling is required for erythropoietin-mediated acute protection against myocardial ischemia/reperfusion injury. Circulation 2004;109:2050–3.

49. Juhaszova M, Zorov DB, Kim SH, et al. Glycogen synthase kinase-3beta mediates convergence of protection signaling to inhibit the mitochondrial permeability transition pore. J Clin Invest 2004;113:1535–49.

50. Shi Y, Rafiee P, Su J, et al. Acute cardioprotective effects of erythropoietin in infant rabbits are mediated by activation of protein kinases and potassium channels. Basic Res Cardiol 2004;99:173–82.

51. Liu X, Xie W, Liu P, et al. Mechanism of the cardioprotection of rhEPO pretreatment on suppressing the inflammatory response in ischemia-reperfusion. Life Sci 2006;78:2255–64.

52. Burger D, Lei M, Geoghegan-Morphet N, et al. Erythropoietin protects cardiomyocytes from apoptosis via up-regulation of endothelial nitric oxide synthase. Cardiovasc Res 2006;72:51–9.

53. Urao N, Okigaki M, Yamada H, et al. Erythropoietin-mobilized endothelial progenitors enhance reendothelialization via Akt-endothelial nitric oxide synthase activation and prevent neointimal hyperplasia. Circ Res 2006;98:1341–3.

54. Vanhoutte PM. The endothelium modulator of vascular smooth-muscle tone. N Engl J Med 1988;319:512–3.

55. Vallance P, Collier J, Moncada S. Effects of endothelium derived nitric oxide on peripheral arteriolar tone in man. Lancet 1989;2:997–1000.

56. Radomski MW, Palmer RM, Moncada S. Endogenous nitric oxide inhibits human platelet adhesion to vascular endothelium. Lancet 1987;2:1057–8.

57. Lindenblatt N, Menger MD, Klar E, et al. Darbepoetin-alpha does not promote microvascular thrombus formation in mice: role of eNOS-dependent protection through platelet and endothelial cell deactivation. Arterioscler Thromb Vasc Biol 2007;27:1191–8.

58. Dubey RK, Jackson EK, Luscher TF. Nitric oxide inhibits angiotensin II-induced migration of rat aortic smooth muscle cells. Role of cyclic-nucleotides and angiotensin 1 receptors. J Clin Invest 1995;96:141–9.

59. Kubes P, Suzuki M, Granger DN. Nitric oxide: an endogenous modulator of leukocyte adhesion. Proc Natl Acad Sci U S A 1991;88:4651–5.

60. Ruschitzka FT, Wenger RH, Stallmach T, et al. Nitric oxide prevents cardiovascular disease and determines survival in polyglobulic mice overexpressing erythropoietin. Proc Natl Acad Sci U S A 2000;97:11609–13.

61. Moon C, Krawczyk M, Ahn D, et al. Erythropoietin reduces myocardial infarction and left ventricular functional decline after coronary artery ligation in rats. Proc Natl Acad Sci U S A 2003;100:11612–7.

62. Parsa CJ, Matsumoto A, Kim J, et al. A novel protective effect of erythropoietin in the infarcted heart. J Clin Invest 2003;112:999–1007.

63. Calvillo L, Latini R, Kajstura J, et al. Recombinant human erythropoietin protects the myocardium from ischemia-reperfusion injury and promotes beneficial remodeling. Proc Natl Acad Sci U S A 2003;100:4802–6.

64. Tada H, Kagaya Y, Takeda M, et al. Endogenous erythropoietin system in non-hematopoietic lineage cells plays a protective role in myocardial ischemia/reperfusion. Cardiovasc Res 2006;71:466–77.

65. Fliser D, de Groot K, Bahlmann FH, et al. Cardiovascular disease in renal patients–a matter of stem cells? Nephrol Dial Transplant 2004;19:2952–4.

66. Bahlmann FH, de Groot K, Haller H, et al. Erythropoietin: is it more than correcting anemia? Nephrol Dial Transplant 2004;19:20–2.

67. Bahlmann FH, De Groot K, Spandau JM, et al. Erythropoietin regulates endothelial progenitor cells. Blood 2004;103:921–6.

68. Bahlmann FH, DeGroot K, Duckert T, et al. Endothelial progenitor cell proliferation and differentiation is regulated by erythropoietin. Kidney Int 2003;64:1648–52.

69. Mangi AA, Noiseux N, Kong D, et al. Mesenchymal stem cells modified with Akt prevent remodeling and restore performance of infarcted hearts. Nat Med 2003;9:1195–201.

70. Hamed S, Barshack I, Luboshits G, et al. Erythropoietin improves myocardial performance in doxorubicin-induced cardiomyopathy. Eur Heart J 2006;27:1876–83.

71. Wald M, Gutnisky A, Borda E, et al. Erythropoietin modified the cardiac action of ouabain in chronically anaemic-uraemic rats. Nephron 1995;71:190–6.

72. Marrero MB, Venema RC, Ma H, et al. Erythropoietin receptor-operated Ca2+ channels: activation by phospholipase C-gamma 1. Kidney Int 1998;53:1259–68.

73. Chong ZZ, Kang JQ, Maiese K. Hematopoietic factor erythropoietin fosters neuroprotection through novel signal transduction cascades. J Cereb Blood Flow Metab 2002;22:503–14.

74. Carlini RG, Alonzo EJ, Dominguez J, et al. Effect of recombinant human erythropoietin on endothelial cell apoptosis. Kidney Int 1999;55:546–53.

75. Wizemann V, Kaufmann J, Kramer W. Effect of erythropoietin on ischemia tolerance in anemic hemodialysis patients with confirmed coronary artery disease. Nephron 1992;62:161–5.

76. Portoles J, Torralbo A, Martin P, et al. Cardiovascular effects of recombinant human erythropoietin in predialysis patients. Am J Kidney Dis 1997;29:541–8.

77. Palazzuoli A, Silverberg DS, Calabrò A, et al. Beta-erythropoietin effects on ventricular remodeling, left and right systolic function, pulmonary pressure, and hospitalizations in patients affected with heart failure and anemia. J Cardiovasc Pharmacol 2009;53:462–7.

78. Palazzuoli A, Silverberg DS, Iovine F, et al. Effects of beta erythropoietin treatment on left ventricular remodeling, systolic function, and B-type natriuretic peptide levels in patients with the cardiorenal anemia syndrome. Am Heart J 2007;154:645.

79. Tramontano AF, Muniyappa R, Black AD, et al. Erythropoietin protects cardiac myocytes from hypoxia-induced apoptosis through an Akt-dependent pathway. Biochem Biophys Res Commun 2003;308:990–4.

80. Lipsic E, Westenbrink BD, van der Meer P, et al. Low-dose erythropoietin improves cardiac function in experimental heart failure without increasing haematocrit. Eur J Heart Fail 2008;10:22–9.

81. Moon C, Krawczyk M, Paik D, et al. Erythropoietin, modified to not stimulate red blood cell production, retains its cardioprotective properties. J Pharmacol Exp Ther 2006;316:999–1005.

82. Fiordaliso F, Chimenti S, Staszewsky L, et al. A nonerythropoietic derivative of erythropoietin protects the myocardium from ischemia-reperfusion injury. Proc Natl Acad Sci U S A 2005;102:2046–51.

83. Fairbanks V, Beutler E. Iron deficiency. In: Beutler E, editor. Williams hematology. 6th edition. New York: McGraw-Hill; 2001. p. 295–304, 447–50.

84. Dunn LL, Rahmanto YS, Richardson DR. Iron uptake and metabolism in the new millennium. Trends Cell Biol 2007;17:93–100.

85. Anderson GJ, Vulpe CD. Mammalian iron transport. Cell Mol Life Sci 2009;66:3241–61.

86. Cairo G, Bernuzzi F, Recalcati S. A precious metal: iron, an essential nutrient for all cells. Genes Nutr 2006;1:25–39.

87. Beard JL. Iron biology in immune function, muscle metabolism and neuronal functioning. J Nutr 2001; 131(Suppl 2):568S–79S.

88. Sutak R, Lesuisse E, Tachezy J, et al. Crusade for iron: iron uptake in unicellular eukaryotes and its significance for virulence. Trends Microbiol 2008; 16:261–8.

89. Wilson MT, Reeder BJ. Oxygen-binding haem proteins. Exp Physiol 2008;93:128–32.

90. Rouault TA, Tong WH. Iron-sulphur cluster biogenesis and mitochondrial iron homeostasis. Nat Rev Mol Cell Biol 2005;6:345–51.

91. Gisbert JP, Gomollon F. An update on iron physiology. World J Gastroenterol 2009;15:4617–26.

92. Haas JD, Brownlie T 4th. Iron deficiency and reduced work capacity: a critical review of the research to determine a causal relationship. J Nutr 2001;131(2S-2):676S–90S.

93. Anker SD, Colet JC, Filippatos G, et al. FAIR-HF Trial Investigators. Ferric carboxymaltose in patients with heart failure and iron deficiency. N Engl J Med 2009;361:2436–48.

94. Okonko DO, Grzeslo A, Witkowski T, et al. Effect of intravenous iron sucrose on exercise tolerance in anemic and nonanemic patients with symptomatic chronic heart failure and iron deficiency FERRIC-HF: a randomized, controlled, observer-blinded trial. J Am Coll Cardiol 2008;51:103–12.

95. Ezekowitz JA, McAlister FA, Armstrong PW. Anemia is common in heart failure and is associated with poor outcomes: insights from a cohort of 12,065 patients with new-onset heart failure. Circulation 2003;107:223–5.

96. Nanas JN, Matsouka C, Karageorgopoulos D, et al. Etiology of anemia in patients with advanced heart failure. J Am Coll Cardiol 2006;48:2485–9.

97. Handelman GJ, Levin NW. Iron and anemia in human biology: a review of mechanisms. Heart Fail Rev 2008;13:393–404.

98. Kemna EH, Tjalsma H, Willems HL, et al. Hepcidin: from discovery to differential diagnosis. Haematologica 2008;93:90–7.

99. Viatte L, Vaulont S. Hepcidin, the iron watcher. Biochimie 2009;91:1223–8.

100. Suzuki H, Toba K, Kato K, et al. Serum hepcidin-20 is elevated during the acute phase of myocardial infarction. Tohoku J Exp Med 2009;218:93–8.

101. Matsumoto M, Tsujino T, Lee-Kawabata M, et al. Iron regulatory hormone hepcidin decreases in chronic heart failure patients with anemia. Circ J 2010;74:301–6.

102. Merle U, Fein E, Gehrke SG, et al. The iron regulatory peptide hepcidin is expressed in the heart and regulated by hypoxia and inflammation. Endocrinology 2007;148:2663–8.

103. Ge XH, Wang Q, Qian ZM, et al. The iron regulatory hormone hepcidin reduces ferroportin 1 content and iron release in H9C2 cardiomyocytes. J Nutr Biochem 2009;20:860–5.

104. Qian ZM, Chang YZ, Leung G, et al. Expression of ferroportin1, hephaestin and ceruloplasmin in rat heart. Biochim Biophys Acta 2007;1772:527–32.

105. Isoda M, Hanawa H, Watanabe R, et al. Expression of the peptide hormone hepcidin increases in cardiomyocytes under myocarditis and myocardial infarction. J Nutr Biochem 2010, in press.

106. Turner LR, Premo DA, Gibbs BJ, et al. Adaptations to iron deficiency: cardiac functional responsiveness to norepinephrine, arterial remodeling, and the effect of beta-blockade on cardiac hypertrophy. BMC Physiol 2002;2:1.

107. Rossi MA, Carillo SV. Electron microscopic study on the cardiac hypertrophy induced by iron deficiency anemia in the rat. Br J Exp Pathol 1983; 64:373–87.

108. Tanne Z, Coleman R, Nahir M, et al. Ultrastructural and cytochemical changes in the heart of iron-deficient rats. Biochem Pharmacol 1994;47:1759–66.

109. Olivetti G, Lagrasta C, Quaini F, et al. Capillary growth in anemia-induced ventricular wall remodeling in the rat heart. Circ Res 1989;65:1182–92.

110. Olivetti G, Quaini F, Lagrasta C, et al. Myocyte cellular hypertrophy and hyperplasia contribute to ventricular wall remodeling in anemia-induced cardiac hypertrophy in rats. Am J Pathol 1992; 141:227–39.

111. Medeiros DM, Beard JL. Dietary iron deficiency results in cardiac eccentric hypertrophy in rats. Proc Soc Exp Biol Med 1998;218:370–5.

112. Dong F, Zhang X, Culver B, et al. Dietary iron deficiency induces ventricular dilation, mitochondrial ultrastructural aberrations and cytochrome *c* release: involvement of nitric oxide synthase and protein tyrosine nitration. Clin Sci 2005;109:277–86.

113. Chvapil M, Hurych J, Ehrlichová E. The effect of iron deficiency on the synthesis of collagenous and non-collagenous proteins in wound granulation tissue and in the heart of rats. Exp Med Surg 1968; 26:52–60.

114. Naito Y, Tsujino T, Matsumoto M, et al. Adaptive response of the heart to long-term anemia induced by iron deficiency. Am J Physiol Heart Circ Physiol 2009;296:H585–593.

Treatment with Iron of Patients with Heart Failure With and Without Anemia

Qurat-ul-ain Jelani, MD[a], Philipp Attanasio, MD[b],
Stuart D. Katz, MD[a], Stefan D. Anker, MD, PhD[b,c],*

KEYWORDS

- Iron deficiency • Anemia • Chronic heart failure
- Intravenous iron

Iron is an essential trace element that plays an important role in many homeostatic processes in the human body. Major physiological functions of iron include oxygen transport, as a component of hemoglobin (Hb) and myoglobin, and maintenance of energy production through oxidative phosphorylation as an integral component of cytochromes, nicotinamide adenine dinucleotide (NADH) and succinate dehydrogenases.[1–3] Iron plays an important role in immune regulation as a component of peroxide- and nitric oxide-generating enzymes required by some immune cells for normal host defenses.[1–3] Iron is also increasingly recognized to be an important transcription factor for a variety of other signal pathways related to cell growth and inflammation.[1–3] Iron deficiency may, therefore, be associated with a variety of symptoms and decreased exercise capacity. Nevertheless, treatment with iron is not free of challenges. Some experimental studies suggest that, in response to iron, reactive oxygen species are generated that could impair cellular function. The authors aim to review the literature focusing on the aspects of iron physiology and biochemistry that may be relevant for chronic heart failure (CHF).

PHYSIOLOGY OF IRON STORAGE AND ITS LABORATORY MEASUREMENT

Total body iron stores are regulated exclusively through control of iron absorption; there are no known natural metabolic pathways for iron excretion.[4] Hepcidin is a liver-derived 25 amino acid peptide hormone that appears to play a critical role in the regulation of iron absorption.[5] The physiological signals that regulate hepcidin secretion are not fully characterized but appear to be related to iron-dependent redox signaling related to pathways involving the HFE, TRF2, and HJV genes; red cell mass; and cytokine signaling.[6] In a negative feedback loop, hepcidin is secreted in response to increased body iron stores and interacts with ferroportin and other iron transport proteins in the enterocyte to inhibit gut iron absorption.[6,7]

Almost all iron is bound to specific iron transport proteins (transferrin) and iron storage proteins (ferritin) in a tightly regulated system that controls iron availability to the bone marrow for erythropoiesis. A small amount of low-molecular weight, nonprotein-bound iron complexed to citrate and other small molecules has also been described in the extracellular and intracellular compartments outside of the reticuloendothelial system.[7,8] In

---

[a] The Leon H. Charney Division of Cardiology, New York University School of Medicine, 530 First Avenue, Skirball- 9R, New York, NY 10016, USA
[b] Department of Cardiology, Charite Medical School, Augustenburger Platz 1, 13353 Berlin, Germany
[c] Centre for Clinical and Basic Research, IRCCS San Raffaele Roma, Via della Pisana, Roma 235 00163, Italy
* Corresponding author. Department of Cardiology, Charité Universitätsmedizin, Augustenburger Platz 1, Berlin 13353, Germany.
E-mail address: s.anker@cachexia.de

Heart Failure Clin 6 (2010) 305–312
doi:10.1016/j.hfc.2010.02.002
1551-7136/10/$ – see front matter © 2010 Elsevier Inc. All rights reserved.

nonheme tissues, two iron regulatory proteins (IRP-1 and IRP-2) play an important role in maintaining intracellular iron homeostasis. In response to changes in iron availability and redox signals, IRP-1 and IRP-2 bind iron-response elements that regulate transcription of transferrin receptor, ferritin, and other proteins.[4,9]

Low molecular weight, nontransferrin-bound iron is present in the serum of normal subjects in concentrations ranging from 0.08 to 0.19 μM. Increased levels of nontransferrin-bound iron have been reported in patients with iron overload secondary to end-stage renal disease, hemolytic anemias, and hemochromatosis.[10] Low molecular weight iron appears to be transported across cell membranes by poorly characterized transporter proteins distinct from the transferrin receptor, as patients with chronic iron overload manifest increased intracellular iron despite downregulation of transferrin receptors.[11] The low molecular weight iron pool is readily chelatable, is available for participation in redox reactions via Fenton chemistry and interactions with nitric oxide, and regulates synthesis and activity of iron-containing proteins.[8,12]

Iron stores in the body may be assessed by a variety of clinically available blood biomarkers. Normal total body iron stores range from 30 to 40 mg/kg body weight, with 1.8 grams contained within red blood cells (depending on blood volume and Hb concentration), and approximately 1.6 gm in storage in liver parenchymal cells and the reticuloendothelial system.[13] Normal daily loss of iron from sloughing of gastrointestinal mucosal cells is approximately 1 to 2 mg/day with losses generally matched by gastrointestinal absorption of an equal amount.[13] Bone marrow iron content is considered the gold standard test for the evaluation of iron stores, but this procedure is invasive and therefore not routinely used in clinical evaluation of anemia. Blood markers of iron stores include total iron-binding capacity (circulating transferrin), serum iron, percent transferrin saturation, plasma ferritin, sideroblast (percent), red blood cell protoporphyrin level, and erythrocyte morphology (**Table 1**). The problem of how to define iron deficiency in heart failure patients is discussed below.

Whereas laboratory assessment of iron stores yield fairly reliable results in most cases with overt signs of iron overload or deficiency, very little data exist on the optimal levels of iron required by the human body for normal physiological function. Available evidence suggests that there may be subclinical states of iron depletion or excess that may be impacting iron-dependent biological processes without overt evidence of iron deficiency or overload.[14,15] This article considers potential implications of this dilemma relevant to evaluation and treatment of iron deficiency in heart failure patients.

ANEMIA IN CHRONIC HEART FAILURE

CHF is characterized by neurohormonal and reflex system activation,[16,17] inflammation,[18] peripheral vasoconstriction,[19] and endocrine metabolic problems,[20] including insulin resistance[21] and cachexia.[22] Anemia is another important comorbidity in this patient population. Its prevalence roughly ranges between 20% and 30%. In the Carvedilol or Metoprolol European Trial (COMET), 29% of the men and 27% of the woman participating developed anemia within the 5 years of follow up.[23] A large study with 12000 new onset heart failure patients showed 17% to be anemic[24] and, in 600 patients hospitalized for acute heart failure, prevalence of anemia was 29%.[25] The cause of anemia in CHF is often difficult to determine and in many cases may be multifactorial. Possible mechanisms include insufficient erythropoietin secretion (due in part to inhibition of the renin angiotensin system) or resistance to the effects of endogenous erythropoietin (due to chronic inflammation), hemodilution, concomitant kidney disease, and iron deficiency.[20,26–32]

Anemia in heart failure patients is associated with increased risk of hospitalization and mortality. Retrospective studies showed a 47% increase in hospitalizations and a 50% to 60% increase in mortality in anemic heart failure patients.[33,34] Anemia also is associated with worse quality of life and it reduces exercise tolerance.[35]

IRON DEFICIENCY IN CHRONIC HEART FAILURE

Iron deficiency in heart failure patients is multifactorial; some of the postulated causes are malnutrition, uremic gastritis, malabsorption due to edematous bowel wall, chronic aspirin or oral anticoagulant use, and abnormal iron mobilization due to cytokine activation.[24,36–38] In a large epidemiological study with more than 12000 new onset heart failure patients, 17% were found to be anemic with 21% of the anemia cases attributable to "iron deficiency."[24] This may be a gross underestimate, as this study was based on International Classification of Diseases reporting, which in itself is based on (1) the physician's thinking about iron deficiency when making the record and (2) the current definition of iron deficiency used in the context of heart failure. Nanas and colleagues[39] determined that 73% of patients with advanced

Table 1
Changes in different iron parameters in states of increased or decreased body iron content

	Normal	Iron Overload	Iron Deficiency Anemia
Marrow iron stores	2–3+	4+	0
Transferrin iron-binding capacity (mcg/dl)	330 ± 30	<300	410
Plasma ferritin (mcg/dl)	100 ± 60	>250	<10
Plasma transferrin receptor	5.5 ± 1.5	5.5	14
Plasma iron (mcg/dl)	115 ± 50	>200	<40
Transferrin saturation (%)	35 ± 15	>60	<10
Sideroblasts (%)	40–60	40–60	<10
Red blood cell protoporphyrin (mcg/dl)	30	30	200
Erythrocytes	Normal	Normal	Microcytic hypochromic

Data from Herbert V. Anemias. In: Paige DM, editor. Clinical nutrition. 2nd edition. St Louis (MO): CV Mosby; 1988. p. 593.

heart failure and anemia had reduced iron stores based on the iron content of bone marrow biopsies.

The presence of chronic inflammation in many CHF patients may mask the diagnosis of iron deficiency anemia. An interesting feature of anemia of chronic disease (including CHF) is the retention of iron within macrophages, thus limiting the availability of iron for erythropoiesis.[40] Inflammatory cytokines like TNF-alpha, Interferon gamma, and IL-6 up-regulate the iron transport protein DMT1, thus increasing iron uptake, and cause iron retention by down-regulating the expression of ferroportin, which is an iron exporter.[41] The same cytokines up-regulate hepcidin, which contributes to iron deficiency and hence anemia of chronic disease, by blocking iron release from macrophages and uptake of iron from the intestinal cells into the blood by interacting with ferroportin.[42,43] These inflammation-related changes in iron metabolism complicate interpretation of clinical tests of iron stores. Weiss and Goodnough[40] suggest that in patients with evidence of inflammation and anemia, with a transferrin saturation less than 16% and ferritin value of less than 30 ng/mL, the diagnosis of absolute iron deficiency anemia can be made. Also, if ferritin is greater than 100 ng/mL, anemia of chronic disease should be the diagnosis. These definitions have not been tested in treatment studies. Anker and colleagues[44] defined presence of functional iron deficiency in CHF based on a ferritin level less than 100 ng/mL, or alternatively when ferritin levels were between 100 and 299 ng/mL, if the transferrin saturation was less than 20%.

The available studies suggest that iron deficiency may be more common than suspected based on analysis of blood markers of iron stores with or without anemia. Subclinical iron deficiency may contribute to the symptoms of the heart failure syndrome, as previous reports indicate that iron deficiency is associated with decreased aerobic capacity independent of the presence of anemia. The mechanisms linking iron deficiency and aerobic capacity have not been fully characterized but may be partly attributable to abnormal oxygen transport in skeletal muscle.

IRON DEFICIENCY AND SYMPTOMS OF HEART FAILURE

Exercise capacity is highly dependent on delivery and utilization of oxygen in active skeletal muscle. In CHF, reduced cardiac output reserve, impaired vasodilatory mechanisms that limit exercise-induced muscle hyperemia, and abnormalities in skeletal muscle mass and metabolism all appear to be important factors in the pathophysiology of exercise intolerance.[45] The major proteins responsible for oxygen transport and transfer (Hb and myoglobin), and oxygen utilization in skeletal muscle (cytochromes and other iron-sulfur enzymes involved in electron transport in mitochondria) all contain iron.[3]

The role of iron deficiency on aerobic capacity has been investigated in animals and human subjects. In rats fed a low iron diet, the reduction of iron in Hb is proportional to the reduction of iron in iron-containing oxidative enzymes in skeletal muscle.[46] In animal models of iron deficiency, maximal aerobic capacity increases in direct proportion to the increase in Hb concentration, but changes in iron-dependent muscle metabolism lagged behind the change in Hb, suggesting that abnormalities in substrate utilization and reduced endurance performance may persist even after correction of Hb.[3,47] Data from human subjects on the relation between iron stores and aerobic capacity are more difficult to interpret, as reduced Hb levels confound interpretation of the direct effects of iron deficiency in skeletal muscle. Nonetheless, some studies suggest that iron deficiency is associated with greater impairment of exercise endurance at submaximal levels even when accounting for decreased oxygen delivery.[3,47] Taken together with the experimental findings in animal models, these findings in human subjects suggest that impaired oxygen utilization in skeletal muscle due to depletion of iron-containing oxidative enzymes may contribute to reduced aerobic capacity associated with iron deficiency.

Several investigators have reported on the effects of iron supplementation in patients with heart failure with and without anemia. The findings of these studies summarized below provide additional data in support of the concept that subclinical iron deficiency without anemia may contribute to reduced aerobic performance in this population.

STUDIES ON THE USE OF PARENTERAL IRON SUPPLEMENTATION IN PATIENTS WITH HEART FAILURE

In a prospective, uncontrolled study, Bolger and colleagues[48] studied the effects of intravenous iron in anemic heart failure patients. Seventeen heart failure patients were enrolled and 16 completed the study. Patients enrolled had systolic heart failure, stable on standard heart failure medication for greater than or equal to 6 weeks and Hb of less than or equal to 12 g/dL. Iron deficiency was defined when ferritin was less than or equal to 400 ng/mL. Patients were given bolus injections of undiluted iron sucrose (200 mg) on days 1, 3, and 5 in an outpatient setting. Serum ferritin was measured on day 12. For patients with a ferritin of less than 400 ng/mL on day 12, further doses were administered on day 15 and 17. At entry, 9 patients were in the New York Heart Association (NYHA) class II symptoms and the remainder in class III. At follow-up, all patients were in NYHA functional class II ($P<.02$). The Minnesota Living with Heart Failure (MLWHF) questionnaire score improved ($P = .02$). The mean 6-minute walk distance increased from 242 ± 78 minutes to 286 ± 72 ($P = .01$). Changes in the latter two correlated strongly with increase in Hb ($R=0.76$, $P = .002$ and $R = 0.56$, $P = .03$,

respectively). Hb, ferritin, serum iron, and transferrin saturation consistently rose from baseline. The investigators reported that the drug was well tolerated.

In a randomized, placebo-controlled study, Toblli and colleagues[49] investigated the effects of iron sucrose on N-terminal pro-brain natriuretic peptide (NT-proBNP) in anemic heart failure patients who also had renal insufficiency (glomerular filtration rate <90 mL/min). Forty patients were enrolled with 20 in the iron sucrose group and 20 in the placebo group. Those enrolled had a left ventricular ejection fraction (LVEF) less than or equal to 35%, NYHA functional class II to IV, anemia with an Hb less than 12.5 g/dL in men and 11.5 g/dL in women, and a serum ferritin less than 100 ng/mL or a transferrin saturation less than or equal to 20%.

Patients in the iron group received intravenous iron sucrose complex weekly for 5 weeks (200 mg/week) and those in the placebo group received isotonic saline, 0.9%. Both groups were followed for a period of 5 months at monthly intervals with patients receiving a further 200 mg of iron every 4 weeks. In patients receiving iron, significant increases were observed in Hb, ferritin, and transferrin saturation and significant reduction observed in NT-proBNP ($P<.001$) and C-reactive protein ($P<.01$) at the end of the study. A significant negative correlation ($P<.01$) between Hb and NT-proBNP at baseline in both groups was observed. The same correlation was observed between Hb and C-reactive protein initially and at the end of study in both groups. Symptomatic improvement was evident by significant changes in NYHA class and MLWHF score ($P<.001$). A reduction in hospitalization rates was also observed in the drug group. There was also an improvement in exercise tolerance compared to baseline and placebo group.

In the Ferric Iron Sucrose in Heart Failure (FERRIC-HF) trial, the effect of intravenous iron sucrose on exercise tolerance in CHF patients was studied.[50] Thirty-five CHF patients were enrolled and randomized in a 2:1 manner (intravenous iron, n = 24, control n = 11). Key eligibility criteria included NYHA functional class II or III symptoms at study entry; exercise limitation characterized by a peak VO$_2$/kg less than or equal to 18 mL/kg/min; Hb concentration of less than 12.5 g/dl for anemic subjects and 12.5 to 14.5 g/dl for nonanemic subjects; serum ferritin of less than 100 ng/mL or between 100 and 299 ng/mL with a transferrin saturation of less than 20%; and an LVEF of less than or equal to 45%. Patients in the intravenous iron group received the drug weekly for 3 to 5 weeks (therapeutic phase, 200 mg iron per week—total dose according to Ganzoni formula) followed by 200 mg doses every 4 weeks to week 16 (maintenance phase). Iron therapy was withheld if ferritin was greater than or equal to 500 ng/mL, Hb was greater than or equal to 16.0 g/dL, or transferrin saturation was greater than or equal to 45% at any stage. The primary endpoint was the change in absolute peak VO_2 from baseline to week 18. Secondary endpoints included changes in peak VO_2 (mL/kg/min) from baseline to week 18 adjusted for body weight, duration of exercise, Hb, and iron studies, as well as changes in NYHA functional class, patient global assessment on a seven-point scale, the MLHF questionnaire score and fatigue score.

Considering the whole population, patients receiving iron sucrose improved in exercise capacity (total peak VO_2 [mL/min]: $P = .08$; weight-adjusted peak VO_2 [mL/kg/min]: $P = .01$). In the anemic group, absolute peak VO_2 significantly improved by 204 mL/min ($P = .02$) and the peak VO2/kg improved by 3.9 mL/kg/min ($P = .009$). Nonanemic patients did not demonstrate the same magnitude of effects. No significant changes in treadmill exercise time were observed in either subgroup alone (overall: $P = .08$). In 44% of patients (n = 8) in the iron group, the NYHA functional class improved. Furthermore, in anemic patients the improvement at week 18 was significant ($P = .048$, 95%, CI −1.0–0). Significant increase in ferritin and transferrin saturation was observed in the iron group in both the anemic and nonanemic group, but did not change in control group. Changes in peak VO_2 were related to changes in transferrin saturation in anemic patients (n = 18, $R = 0.62$, $P = .006$). The investigators concluded that, in patients with CHF and functional iron deficiency, intravenous iron is associated with significant improvements in maximal exercise capacity and accompanied by improved symptoms. The improvements were more pronounced in anemic than nonanemic patients, but one needs to consider that the inclusion was up to a Hb value of 14.5 g/dL, which is higher than in the Ferinject Assessment in Patients With Iron Deficiency and Chronic Heart Failure (FAIR-HF) study where the limit was 13.5 g/dL.

Usmanov and colleagues[51] studied the effects of intravenous iron in 32 anemic patients with moderate to severe CHF and chronic renal insufficiency. The variables studied were hematological parameters, functional status, and cardiac function as assessed by echocardiogram. Thirty-two CHF patients with Hb less than 11 g/dL, NYHA functional class III or IV with a serum creatinine less than 4 mg/dL were enrolled. One-hundred

mg intravenous iron sucrose (Venofer) was administered three times weekly for 3 weeks followed by once weekly for 23 weeks (total dose of 3200 mg). At the end of the study, 9 of the 19 NYHA functional class III improved to class II (47.4%, $P<.01$). However, none of the patients in NYHA IV demonstrated improvement in functional capacity. Echocardiographic parameters, including posterior wall thickness, left ventricular mass index, septal thickness, left ventricular end diastolic volume, and end systolic volume, showed a significant improvement. All hematological parameters in both NYHA III and IV also showed a significant increase over the 6 months treatment period.

In a multicenter, randomized, placebo-controlled, double-blind prospective study Anker and colleagues[44] investigated the effects of ferric carboxymaltose (FCM) in CHF patients with iron deficiency, with or without anemia. In the FAIR-HF trial, 459 patients with CHF were enrolled in a 2:1 ratio: 304 were assigned to receive FCM while 155 received placebo. Key inclusion criteria included NYHA functional class II or III, LVEF less than or equal to 40% (in patients with NYHA class II), or less than or equal to less than or equal to 45% (for NYHA class III), and presence of functional iron deficiency (defined as detailed before by a ferritin <100 ng/mL or ferritin 100–299 ng/mL with transferrin saturation <20%). The screening Hb value had to be between 9.5 g/dL and 13.5 g/dL. Anemia was defined by an Hb less than or equal to 12.0 g/dL at baseline. An intravenous bolus injection of 200 mg FCM or placebo was followed by weekly doses (correction phase; total dose calculated according to Ganzoni formula) and then every 4 weeks (maintenance phase) until week 24. Study drug was administered in a double-blind manner. The coprimary endpoints were self-reported patient global assessment (PGA) and NYHA functional class at week 24. Secondary endpoints included the aforementioned at weeks 4 and 12, plus the distance on the 6 minute walk test and the overall score on the Kansas City Cardiomyopathy Questionnaire and the European Quality of Life-5 Dimensions at weeks 4, 12, and 24. Safety endpoints were serious and nonserious adverse events, hospitalizations, and death assessed up to week 26.

For the study primary endpoints, 50% of patients in the intravenous iron group reported moderate-to-much improvement on the PGA compared to 27% in the placebo group (odds ratio 2.51; 95%CI, 1.75–3.61; $P<.001$) at week 24. Likewise, 47% showed an improvement in NYHA class I or II compared to 30% in the placebo group (odds ratio 2.40, 95%CI 1.55–3.71; $P<.001$). The secondary endpoints determined at weeks 4 and 12 also showed significant improvement (all $P<.001$). Also, 6-minute walk test distances and quality of life assessments improved significantly ($P<.001$ at 4, 12, and 24 weeks for all comparisons). The results were consistent for all 10 prespecified study subgroups (P value for interaction: $P \geq .10$ for all tests). Of particular importance is that the results were similar in patients with and without anemia (P value for interaction for PGA: 0.98; for NYHA class: 0.51).

The rate of adverse events was similar for both groups. However, the rate of first hospitalization for cardiovascular events in the IV iron group was on the lower side (hazard ratio 0.53; 95%, CI 0.25–1.09; $P = .08$). In terms of side effects, gastrointestinal side effects were more common in the FCM group than in patients on placebo, but this was within the expected range. No anaphylactic reactions were observed and, in six cases, injection-site reaction or a discoloration was reported in the course of the approximately 3000 injections provided during the study. The mean difference between the two study groups for ferritin, transferrin saturation, and Hb was significant at week 24. For ferritin, the difference was 246 plus or minus 20 ng/mL, for Hb, 0.59 plus or minus 0.15 g/dL (all $P<.001$).

In conclusion, this study demonstrated a beneficial effect of intravenous iron therapy on symptoms, physical performance, and quality of life for patients with CHF with and without anemia. From a pathophysiological standpoint, the study cannot determine how the observed benefits are achieved, but the findings are consistent with the hypothesis linking iron deficiency and changes in skeletal muscle oxidative capacity. Also, the study duration is too short to make definite statements about safety. Further studies to this end are needed.

SUMMARY

There are accumulating data indicating that short-term administration of intravenous iron is associated with improved symptoms and quality of life of patients with heart failure. Initial reports suggest that functional iron deficiency may occur frequently in CHF patients and may contribute to symptoms related to reduced exercise capacity. Further work is needed to more accurately characterize iron stores in the heart failure population and determine the mechanisms of benefit and long-term outcomes associated with supplemental iron therapy.

REFERENCES

1. Failla ML. Trace elements and host defense: recent advances and continuing challenges. J Nutr 2003; 133(5 Suppl 1):1443S–7S.
2. Gordeuk VR, Bacon BR, Brittenham GM. Iron overload: causes and consequences. Annu Rev Nutr 1987;7:485–508.
3. Beard JL. Iron biology in immune function, muscle metabolism and neuronal functioning. J Nutr 2001; 131(2S-2):568S–79S [discussion: 80S].
4. Beutler E. Cell biology. "Pumping" iron: the proteins. Science 2004;306(5704):2051–3.
5. Ganz T. Hepcidin, a key regulator of iron metabolism and mediator of anemia of inflammation. Blood 2003;102(3):783–8.
6. Swinkels DW, Janssen MC, Bergmans J, et al. Hereditary hemochromatosis: genetic complexity and new diagnostic approaches. Clin Chem 2006; 52(6):950–68.
7. Hider RC. Nature of nontransferrin-bound iron. Eur J Clin Invest 2002;32(Suppl 1):50–4.
8. Richardson DR, Ponka P. The molecular mechanisms of the metabolism and transport of iron in normal and neoplastic cells. Biochim Biophys Acta 1997;1331(1):1–40.
9. Meyron-Holtz EG, Ghosh MC, Rouault TA. Mammalian tissue oxygen levels modulate iron-regulatory protein activities in vivo. Science 2004;306(5704): 2087–90.
10. Breuer W, Hershko C, Cabantchik ZI. The importance of non-transferrin bound iron in disorders of iron metabolism. Transfus Sci 2000;23(3): 185–92.
11. Pietrangelo A. Physiology of iron transport and the hemochromatosis gene. Am J Physiol Gastrointest Liver Physiol 2002;282(3):G403–14.
12. Ponka P. Cellular iron metabolism. Kidney Int Suppl 1999;69:S2–11.
13. Andrews NC. Disorders of iron metabolism. N Engl J Med 1999;341(26):1986–95.
14. Sullivan JL. Is stored iron safe? J Lab Clin Med 2004; 144(6):280–4.
15. Zheng H, Cable R, Spencer B, et al. Iron stores and vascular function in voluntary blood donors. Arterioscler Thromb Vasc Biol 2005;25(8):1577–83.
16. Ponikowski P, Chua TP, Anker SD, et al. Peripheral chemoreceptor hypersensitivity: an ominous sign in patients with chronic heart failure. Circulation 2001; 104(5):544–9.
17. Leyva F, Anker SD, Egerer K, et al. Hyperleptinaemia in chronic heart failure. Relationships with insulin. Eur Heart J 1998;19(10):1547–51.
18. von Haehling S, Jankowska EA, Anker SD. Tumour necrosis factor-alpha and the failing heart–pathophysiology and therapeutic implications. Basic Res Cardiol 2004;99(1):18–28.

19. Anker SD, Volterrani M, Egerer KR, et al. Tumour necrosis factor alpha as a predictor of impaired peak leg blood flow in patients with chronic heart failure. QJM 1998;91(3):199–203.

20. Anker SD, Volterrani M, Pflaum CD, et al. Acquired growth hormone resistance in patients with chronic heart failure: implications for therapy with growth hormone. J Am Coll Cardiol 2001;38(2):443–52.

21. Doehner W, Rauchhaus M, Ponikowski P, et al. Impaired insulin sensitivity as an independent risk factor for mortality in patients with stable chronic heart failure. J Am Coll Cardiol 2005; 46(6):1019–26.

22. von Haehling S, Lainscak M, Springer J, et al. Cardiac cachexia: a systematic overview. Pharmacol Ther 2009;121(3):227–52.

23. Komajda M, Anker SD, Charlesworth A, et al. The impact of new onset anaemia on morbidity and mortality in chronic heart failure: results from COMET. Eur Heart J 2006;27(12):1440–6.

24. Ezekowitz JA, McAlister FA, Armstrong PW. Anemia is common in heart failure and is associated with poor outcomes: insights from a cohort of 12 065 patients with new-onset heart failure. Circulation 2003;107(2):223–5.

25. von Haehling S, Schefold JE, Mejc-Hodoscek L. Anemia in patients hospitalized for acute heart failure. Clin Res Cardiol, in press.

26. Silverberg DS, Wexler D, Iaina A. The importance of anemia and its correction in the management of severe congestive heart failure. Eur J Heart Fail 2002;4(6):681–6.

27. Torre-Amione G, Bozkurt B, Deswal A, et al. An overview of tumor necrosis factor alpha and the failing human heart. Curr Opin Cardiol 1999;14(3):206–10.

28. Sharma R, Anker SD. Cytokines, apoptosis and cachexia: the potential for TNF antagonism. Int J Cardiol 2002;85(1):161–71.

29. Kalra PR, Anagnostopoulos C, Bolger AP, et al. The regulation and measurement of plasma volume in heart failure. J Am Coll Cardiol 2002;39(12):1901–8.

30. Anand IS, Chandrashekhar Y, Ferrari R, et al. Pathogenesis of oedema in chronic severe anaemia: studies of body water and sodium, renal function, haemodynamic variables, and plasma hormones. Br Heart J 1993;70(4):357–62.

31. Chatterjee B, Nydegger UE, Mohacsi P. Serum erythropoietin in heart failure patients treated with ACE-inhibitors or AT(1) antagonists. Eur J Heart Fail 2000;2(4):393–8.

32. Ishani A, Weinhandl E, Zhao Z, et al. Angiotensin-converting enzyme inhibitor as a risk factor for the development of anemia, and the impact of incident anemia on mortality in patients with left ventricular dysfunction. J Am Coll Cardiol 2005;45(3):391–9.

33. Sharma R, Francis DP, Pitt B, et al. Haemoglobin predicts survival in patients with chronic heart failure: a substudy of the ELITE II trial. Eur Heart J 2004;25(12):1021–8.

34. Mozaffarian D, Nye R, Levy WC. Anemia predicts mortality in severe heart failure: the prospective randomized amlodipine survival evaluation (PRAISE). J Am Coll Cardiol 2003;41(11):1933–9.

35. Kalra PR, Bolger AP, Francis DP, et al. Effect of anemia on exercise tolerance in chronic heart failure in men. Am J Cardiol 2003;91(7):888–91.

36. Witte KK, Desilva R, Chattopadhyay S, et al. Are hematinic deficiencies the cause of anemia in chronic heart failure? Am Heart J 2004;147(5): 924–30.

37. Westenbrink BD, Voors AA, van Veldhuisen DJ. Is anemia in chronic heart failure caused by iron deficiency? J Am Coll Cardiol 2007;49(23):2301–2 [author reply: 2].

38. Berry C, Norrie J, Hogg K, et al. The prevalence, nature, and importance of hematologic abnormalities in heart failure. Am Heart J 2006;151(6): 1313–21.

39. Nanas JN, Matsouka C, Karageorgopoulos D, et al. Etiology of anemia in patients with advanced heart failure. J Am Coll Cardiol 2006;48(12):2485–9.

40. Weiss G, Goodnough LT. Anemia of chronic disease. N Engl J Med 2005;352(10):1011–23.

41. Ludwiczek S, Aigner E, Theurl I, et al. Cytokine-mediated regulation of iron transport in human monocytic cells. Blood 2003;101(10):4148–54.

42. Nemeth E, Tuttle MS, Powelson J, et al. Hepcidin regulates cellular iron efflux by binding to ferroportin and inducing its internalization. Science 2004; 306(5704):2090–3.

43. Nemeth E, Rivera S, Gabayan V, et al. IL-6 mediates hypoferremia of inflammation by inducing the synthesis of the iron regulatory hormone hepcidin. J Clin Invest 2004;113(9):1271–6.

44. Anker SD, Comin Colet J, Filippatos G, et al. Ferric carboxymaltose in patients with heart failure and iron deficiency. N Engl J Med 2009;361(25): 2436–48.

45. Katz SD, Zheng H. Peripheral limitations of maximal aerobic capacity in patients with chronic heart failure. J Nucl Cardiol 2002;9(2):215–25.

46. Haas JD, Brownlie T 4th. Iron deficiency and reduced work capacity: a critical review of the research to determine a causal relationship. J Nutr 2001;131(2S-2):676S–88S [discussion: 88S–90S].

47. Davies KJ, Maguire JJ, Brooks GA, et al. Muscle mitochondrial bioenergetics, oxygen supply, and work capacity during dietary iron deficiency and repletion. Am J Physiol 1982;242(6):E418–427.

48. Bolger AP, Bartlett FR, Penston HS, et al. Intravenous iron alone for the treatment of anemia in patients with chronic heart failure. J Am Coll Cardiol 2006;48(6):1225–7.

49. Toblli JE, Lombrana A, Duarte P, et al. Intravenous iron reduces NT-pro-brain natriuretic peptide in anemic patients with chronic heart failure and renal insufficiency. J Am Coll Cardiol 2007;50(17): 1657–65.

50. Okonko DO, Grzeslo A, Witkowski T, et al. Effect of intravenous iron sucrose on exercise tolerance in anemic and nonanemic patients with symptomatic chronic heart failure and iron deficiency FERRIC-HF: a randomized, controlled, observer-blinded trial. J Am Coll Cardiol 2008;51(2):103–12.

51. Usmanov RI, Zueva EB, Silverberg DS, et al. Intravenous iron without erythropoietin for the treatment of iron deficiency anemia in patients with moderate to severe congestive heart failure and chronic kidney insufficiency. J Nephrol 2008;21(2):236–42.

Erythropoiesis Stimulation in Acute Ischemic Syndromes

Willem-Peter T. Ruifrok, MD*, Erik Lipšic, MD, PhD,
Rudolf A. de Boer, MD, PhD, Wiek H. van Gilst, PhD,
Dirk J. van Veldhuisen, MD, PhD

KEYWORDS

- Erythropoietin • Myocardial infarction
- Acute coronary syndrome • Ischemia-reperfusion injury

Erythropoietin (EPO) is a hematopoietic hormone with extensive nonhematopoietic properties. EPO was discovered in 1957[1]; 50 years earlier, in 1906, Carnot and DeFlandre suggested the existence of a circulating erythropoietic factor.[2] At the time of discovery of EPO, the kidneys were established as the predominant side of production. The production of EPO is regulated by hypoxia and is under the control of hypoxia-inducible factor-1.[3] Tissue oxygen demand and oxygen transport capacity regulate endogenous EPO production and secretion.[4,5] EPO stimulates red blood cell production by prevention of physiologic apoptosis, which adds to hematopoietic progenitor cell turnover and increased release of red blood cells into the blood.[6]

The recombinant human form of EPO has provided a breakthrough in the treatment of anemia caused mostly by EPO deficiency in chronic kidney disease. The use of EPO has markedly increased in the last decades and is now widely applied in cancer patients receiving chemotherapy, HIV-positive patients, treatment of myelodysplastic syndromes, and as prophylaxis to reduce blood transfusions during major surgery.

A functional EPO receptor (EPOR), which was previously thought only to be present in hematopoietic progenitor cells, is also expressed in nonhematopoietic systems, such as the cardiovascular system and the central nervous system.[7] These discoveries fuelled intense research into the nonhematopoietic effects of EPO.

EPO modulates a broad array of cellular processes that include progenitor stem cell development, cellular integrity, and angiogenesis (**Fig. 1**). EPO is emerging as a cell death blocker and a vascular growth factor with promising protective potential in the setting of acute and chronic myocardial ischemia and may potentially represent a powerful pharmacologic addendum in the fight against cardiovascular diseases. This article provides an overview of the use of erythropoiesis-stimulating agents in acute myocardial ischemia.

EPO-EPOR SYSTEM AND ISCHEMIA: EVIDENCE FROM ANIMAL EXPERIMENTAL STUDIES

Expression of EPOR has been shown in numerous tissues, including the reproductive organs, liver, kidneys, endothelial and vascular smooth cells, brain, and the heart.[5,8–17] EPOR is a member of the type 1 cytokine receptor family characterized by a single transmembrane domain.[18] Under normal circumstances EPO and EPOR have a relatively low expression in nonhematopoietic tissue[19]; however, expression of EPO and EPOR is rapidly increased in response to hypoxia and a number of other metabolic stressors including proinflammatory cytokines, hypoglycemia, and

Department of Cardiology, University Medical Center Groningen, University of Groningen, PO Box 30.001, 9700 RB Groningen, The Netherlands
* Corresponding author.
E-mail address: w.t.ruifrok@thorax.umcg.nl

Heart Failure Clin 6 (2010) 313–321
doi:10.1016/j.hfc.2009.12.002
1551-7136/10/$ – see front matter © 2010 Elsevier Inc. All rights reserved.

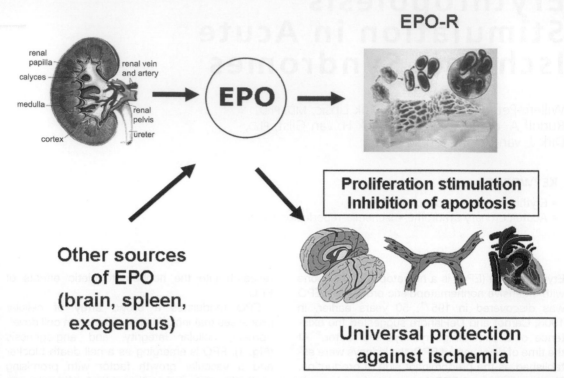

Fig. 1. Biologic functions of erythropoietin (EPO): classical hematopoietic and nonhematopoietic effects of EPO.

increased reactive oxygen species.[4,5,14] These stressors directly activate the hypoxia-inducible factor pathways, which in turn regulate the gene transcription of EPO and EPOR.[20,21] Activation of EPOR leads to downstream activation of intracellular pathways, such as phosphatidylinositol 3-kinase/Akt (PI3K/Akt), extracellular signal-regulated kinases 1/2 (ERK1/2), and signal transducers and activators of transcription (STAT) (Fig. 2). These pathways are associated with cell survival.[22–26] These pathways originate with the binding of EPO to EPOR to activate Janus kinase 2 (Jak2).[9,24] Subsequently, PI3K and Akt are activated by downstream phosphorylation.[27] Activation of the specific gene product STAT5 can regulate EPO-mediated cell proliferation and protect against apoptosis, which are direct substrates of Jak2. EPO maintains cellular integrity and prevents apoptosis through a number of pathways, such as the modulation of apoptosis protease activating factor-1, the release of cytochrome *c*, and the prevention of activation of caspases 9 and 3.[28,29] EPO also modulates cellular inflammation by inhibiting cellular phosphatidyl-serine membrane exposure and subsequent targeting of cells for phagocytosis.[30–32] As a result of upregulation of EPOR (eg, during ischemia), EPO robustly protects the cell, mainly by inhibiting the apoptotic mechanisms of injury.[9]

Genetically engineered mice provided more in-depth insight into the importance of EPOR. EPOR expression in the erythropoietic lineage cells is necessary for normal development of mammals. EPOR knock-out mice, lacking EPOR in their erythroid lineage, die of severe anemia between embryonic day 13 and 15.[33–35] EPO and EPOR play an essential role in proliferation, survival, and differentiation of erythroid progenitor cells.[33,34] Wu and colleagues[36] demonstrated that EPO and EPOR have a major function in embryonic heart development, because EPO$^{-/-}$ and EPOR$^{-/-}$ mice experience ventricular hypoplasia and defects in the intraventricular septum. In addition to these findings, Suzuki and colleagues[37] developed a mouse model in which EPOR expression is restricted to the erythropoietic lineage, by targeted knock-in of the EPOR gene ligated to the GATA-1 promotor, a transcription factor exclusive to erythroid lineage cells (EPOR$^{-/-}$rescued). These mice express EPOR exclusively in their erythropoietic cells, whereas other organs lack EPOR. These mice develop normally and are fertile, so that it seems that EPO and EPOR are dispensable for normal development. When these mice were subjected to various acute and chronic models of cardiovascular disease, however, EPO and EPOR seemed to play a major role in protection against cardiovascular damage. A deficiency

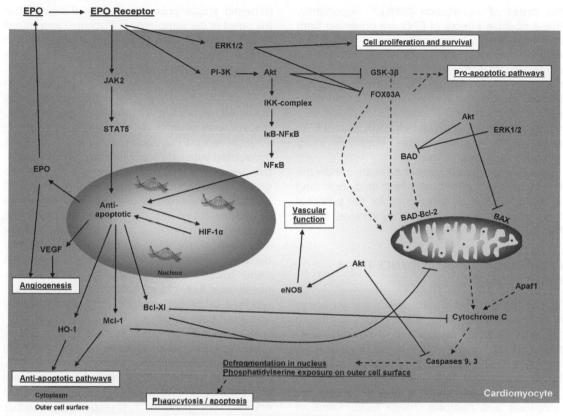

Fig. 2. Overview of the potential mechanisms of cytoprotection of erythropoietin (EPO). Activation of the erythropoietin receptor (EPOR) by EPO leads to downstream activation of intracellular pathways, such as PI3K/akt, ERK1/2, and STAT. These pathways originate with the binding of EPO to the EPOR to activate JAK2. Subsequently, PI3K and Akt are activated by downstream phosphorylation. Activation of STAT can regulate EPO-mediated cell protection and protect against apoptosis. EPO maintains cellular integrity and prevents apoptosis through a number of pathways, such as the modulation of apoptosis protease activating factor-1, the release of cytochrome c, and the prevention of activation of caspases 9 and 3. Dotted lines, suppressed pathways; solid lines, activated pathways.

of the endogenous EPO-EPOR system deteriorates cardiomyocyte survival after ischemia-reperfusion injury and subsequent left ventricular remodeling.[38] This effect is partially caused by enhanced apoptosis of cardiomyocytes.[38–40] Molecular studies in this model suggested that the vascular endothelial growth factor–vascular endothelial growth factor receptor system may be involved in mediating these effects of EPO.[41] Together, current evidence supports a pivotal role of EPOR in the complex cascades of acute hypoxic damage in the body and, more specifically, the cardiovascular system.

In several experimental studies it has been established that EPO exerts cytoprotective effects.[22,42–50] The antiapoptotic effect of EPO is the acute protecting mechanism of EPO during ischemia.[48,51] This effect is independent from hematocrit-increasing effects of EPO, but is rather exerted by distinct apoptotic pathways

(see **Fig. 2**). EPO exerts its potent antiapoptotic effects in a number of cellular systems, including cultured endothelial cells and neonatal rat cardiomyocytes.[9,46] Cavillo and colleagues[52] administered a high-dose of EPO (5000 IU/kg) for 7 consecutive days in an ischemia-reperfusion (I-R) injury model in rats. This reduced cardiomyocyte loss by 50%, an extent sufficient to normalize hemodynamic function within 1 week after reperfusion. Other experimental in vivo studies using an I-R injury model showed decreased infarct size,[26,48,49,53–55] enhancement of left ventricular function,[49,53] and reduced apoptosis,[22,55] even when EPO was administered after the onset of reperfusion.[48] The authors have shown a 16% reduction in number of apoptotic cells in pretreated animals with EPO in an I-R injury model.[48,56] Furthermore, apoptosis was significantly attenuated in animals treated with EPO at the start of ischemia (29% reduction) and after the onset of reperfusion (38%).[48] Importantly, these positive effects of EPO are observed both at a high-dose administration and at a low-dose administration of EPO.[48,54] Nonhematopoietic derivatives of EPO, such as carbamylated EPO, do not have the possible side effects of increased hematocrit, but do have the beneficial nonhematopoietic effects of EPO. Fiordaliso and colleagues[57] showed that a nonerythropoietic derivative of EPO protects the cardiomyocytes from I-R injury without increasing hematocrit.

All of the previously mentioned studies show the beneficial effect of EPO administration, indicating a broad window of opportunity for the potential treatment of acute coronary syndromes in the human setting.

EPO AND ISCHEMIA: EVIDENCE FROM CLINICAL STUDIES

The 1980s and 1990s witnessed a golden age in clinical cardiology trials. Their results led to an unprecedented decrease in mortality and morbidity among patients with acute myocardial infarction (MI), leaving only a limited space for further therapeutic interventions.

The major determinants of final infarct size are apoptosis and necrosis. These major forms of cell death extensively contribute to the extent of damage after an ischemic myocardial event.[58,59] Reperfusion, either by primary coronary intervention or thrombolysis, is a cornerstone of acute MI treatment. Although salvaging the ischemic myocardium, opening the vessel itself may cause another kind of damage called "reperfusion injury[60]." This reperfusion can make up to 50% of the final damage size.[61] Moreover, some patients experience a significant time delay before receiving adequate therapy and hence are prone to develop ischemic cardiomyopathy and heart failure in the long term. Experimental studies suggest a beneficial role of EPO on both limiting the reperfusion injury and late post-MI remodeling.

Although one could argue whether the fast application of experimental results into clinical research is always beneficial, in the case of EPO it was "forcing an open door." EPO is used in clinical medicine since the 1980s, mainly as substitution therapy in patients with end-stage kidney disease. It was only obvious that first clinical studies using EPO for "nonhematopoietic" indications would not take long.

Because of the discovery of the extensive neuroprotective effects of EPO in preclinical studies, the first clinical trials were conducted in various neuropsychiatric disorders. In a randomized, double-blind trial, EPO was given to patients with ischemic stroke presenting within 8 hours after the onset of the symptoms.[62] Patients randomized to EPO group showed significant improvement in clinical outcome parameters, together with decrease in S100β level, a brain damage marker. Also, a strong trend for reduction in infarct size in EPO group as compared with controls was observed. In another randomized, double-blind, placebo-controlled study in patients with chronic schizophrenia, EPO treatment for 3 months was associated with significant improvement in cognitive performance compared with placebo-treated group.[63] Recently, Cariou and colleagues[64] studied the neuroprotective effect of high-dose EPO after out-of-hospital cardiac arrest. In this matched control study survival rates and rates of full neurologic recovery did not differ significantly between EPO-treated patients and controls. A trend toward better neurologic outcome was observed in EPO group, however, which was outweighed by higher incidence of thrombocytosis and thrombotic events.

Nevertheless, all these studies regarded only a very limited amount of patients (around 40–50) and are proof-of-concept trials. The German Multicenter EPO Stroke Trial was designed to evaluate the efficacy and safety of EPO in stroke and enrolled 522 patients.[65] Unexpectedly, neither primary nor secondary outcome parameters showed favorable effects of EPO. It even raised some safety concerns, particularly in patients receiving thrombolysis, with an overall death rate of 16.4% in the EPO and 9% in the placebo group (odds ratio, 1.98; 95% confidence interval, 1.16–3.38; $P = .01$).

The very first feasibility and safety study in patients with acute MI was performed by the authors' group (**Table 1**).[66] In this single-center, investigator-initiated, prospective study 22 patients with first ST-elevation MI were randomized to one bolus darbepoietin alfa (Aranesp) (300 μg) or placebo before undergoing primary percutaneous coronary intervention (PCI). No adverse events were recorded during 30-day follow-up. Left ventricular ejection fraction (LVEF) after 4 months was similar in both groups, as measured by planar radionuclide ventriculography. Although hematocrit levels were not significantly different in both groups, darbepoietin treatment significantly increased the amount of endothelial progenitor cells (CD34+/CD45-).

Interestingly, high levels of endogenous EPO were an independent predictor for the cumulative creatinin kinase release in patients with first MI who received successful primary PCI.[73] In this study, patients with higher endogenous EPO levels were found to have smaller infarcts, suggesting

Table 1
Overview of clinical cardiology studies using EPO as a cytoprotective agent

Study	Study Design	Number Patients	Patients Characteristics	Results
Lipsic et al[66]	Investigator-initiated, prospective feasibility and safety study	22	First ST-elevation MI treated with primary PCI	Darbepoetin administration safe and well tolerated Darbepoetin treatment stimulates EPC mobilization
Liem et al[67]	Prospective, randomized, placebo-controlled study	51	Non-ST elevation MI	No significant effect on enzymatic infarct size
Cleland et al[68]	Prospective, randomized, double-blind, and placebo controlled trial	138	First ST-elevation MI treated with primary PCI	No difference in left ventricular function or infarct size
Binbrek et al[69]	Prospective, randomized, open label, blinded end point trial	236	ST-elevation MI treated with tenecteplase	EPO administration safe, but no enhanced preservation of jeopardized ischemic myocardium
Tanq et al[70]	Prospective, randomized, placebo controlled, double-blind trial	44	Acute MI treated with aspirin and clopidogrel after successful PCI	No alteration of markers of platelet and endothelial cell activation associated with thrombosis Increase in expression of angiogenesis signaling proteins in PBMCs (EPOR, VEGFR-1, p-PI3K)
HEBE III[71]	Prospective, randomized, placebo controlled, open label, blinded end point trial	466	First ST-elevation MI treated with primary PCI	Results are awaited
REVEAL[72]	Prospective, randomized, double-blinded, placebo-controlled study	210	First ST-elevation MI treated with primary PCI	Results are awaited

Abbreviations: EPC, endothelial progenitor cell; EPO, erythropoietin; EPOR, erythropoietin receptor; MI, myocardial infarction; PBMC, peripheral blood mononuclear cell; PCI, percutaneous coronary intervention; p-PI3K, phosphorylated phosphatidylinositol 3-kinase; VEGFR-1, vascular endothelial growth factor receptor 1.

a possible protective mechanism of EPO against I-R injury.

A study by Liem and colleagues[67] evaluated the effect of EPO treatment in patients with non-ST elevation MI. Here, 51 patients were randomized to single intravenous dose of 40,000 IU EPO or a placebo within 8 hours after elevated levels of troponin-I were available. The primary end point of the study, enzymatic infarct size, was not different between the two groups. Both groups had similar event rates up to more than 1 year. Yet, systolic blood pressure in the patients treated with EPO increased significantly in the first hours after onset of EPO therapy compared with placebo controls.

Recently, results of REVIVAL-3, the first prospective, randomized, double-blind, and placebo-controlled trial of EPO in patients with ST-elevation MI were presented.[68] Patients with first acute ST-elevation MI treated with primary PCI and having angiographically LVEF less than 50% were eligible to participate. The patients were randomized to receive 30,000 IU of EPO or placebo during PCI. Study medication was repeated on day 2 and 3. Primary end point of the study was LVEF at 6 months as assessed by MRI. In both groups there was no difference in primary end point, with a similar LVEF at 6 months (52%). Importantly, the secondary end point consisting of combined clinical events (death, recurrent MI, infarct-related artery revascularization, or stroke) occurred in 13% of EPO-treated patients as compared with 5.7% in the placebo group. Although this difference did not reach statistical significance, these possibly serious adverse events could raise concerns about the safety profile of EPO in patients with MI.

A fourth clinical trial with EPO evaluated whether EPO administration early after onset of ischemia could enhance the preservation of jeopardized myocardium by reperfusion (tenecteplase <6 hours after onset of chest pain).[69] Patients were randomized to standard care or standard care plus a single dose of EPO (30,000 IU β-EPO). Although early administration of EPO was safe, the primary end point, enzymatically estimated infarct size, was not different between the two groups.

To assess safety and efficacy markers relevant to the biologic activity of EPO, Tang and colleagues[70] conducted a prospective, placebo-controlled, randomized, double-blind trial to determine the effects of EPO administration (200 μ/kg daily for 3 consecutive days) on different measures of platelet activation platelet and endothelial cell activation, soluble Fas ligand, and peripheral blood mononuclear cell expression of angiogenesis–signaling proteins. Short-term administration of EPO did not alter markers of platelet and endothelial cell activation associated with thrombosis, such as bleeding time, platelet function assay closure time, and von Willebrand factor levels. EPO administration increased expression of angiogenesis signaling proteins in peripheral blood mononuclear cells, however, such as

EPOR, vascular endothelial growth factor receptor-1, and phosphorylated PI3K, indicating biologic activity of EPO administration.

Currently, there are two larger-scale clinical trials in progress (HEBE III and REVEAL) evaluating the effect of EPO in ST-elevation MI. The HEBE III is a multicenter, prospective, randomized, and open-label trial with blinded end points (NCT00449488).[71] The objective is to evaluate the effect of single-bolus EPO administration after a successful PCI for a first ST-elevation MI. The primary end point of the study is the LVEF, measured by planar radionuclide ventriculography. Secondary end points are effects on myocardial infarct size and cardiovascular events. The results of this study are expected at the beginning of 2010.

The second study, REVEAL, is a randomized, double-blinded, placebo-controlled study that evaluates the effects of EPO administration on infarct size, left ventricular remodeling, and circulating endothelial progenitor cells in patients with large MI (NCT00378352).[72] Eligible patients who present to the hospital with an acute ST-elevation MI are randomly assigned to receive a single infusion of study medication consisting either of EPO or placebo. The size of the infarction and the dimensions of the heart are assessed by cardiac MRI within 2 to 6 days of the infusion of the study medication, and again approximately 3 months later. The results of these two studies should give definite answer on the efficacy of EPO treatment in patients with acute MI.

SUMMARY

There is an ongoing discussion about possible discrepancy between preclinical and clinical effects of EPO on the cardiovascular system. Numerous clinical studies of anemia correction by EPO in patients with chronic renal failure raised concerns associated with increased cardiovascular mortality and morbidity.[74,75] It seems that chronic treatment with higher doses, associated with hematocrit increase, could also lead to potential adverse effect, such as thrombocytosis and activation of endothelium. This is of particular importance in patients undergoing PCI with stent implantation and prone to stent thrombosis.

The tissue protective effect of EPO seems independent, however, of its hematopoietic activity. Low-dose EPO treatment led to vascular and cardiac protection without raising hematocrit.[76,77] Another possibility to avoid EPO side effects could be using variants of EPO without hematopoietic activity, which retain antiapoptotic and angiogenetic properties.[57,78] The future of EPO within cardiology presumably lies in the development of and applying nonhematopoietic EPO derivates in the treatment of acute coronary syndromes. The final verdict on EPO treatment for acute coronary syndromes will soon be pronounced; however the search for cellular protection against ischemia continues regardless of these results.

REFERENCES

1. Jacobson LO, Goldwasser E, Fried W, et al. Role of the kidney in erythropoiesis. Nature 1957;179(4560): 633–4.

2. Erslev AJ. Erythropoietin. N Engl J Med 1991; 324(19):1339–44.

3. Fandrey J. Oxygen-dependent and tissue-specific regulation of erythropoietin gene expression. Am J Physiol Regul Integr Comp Physiol 2004;286(6): R977–88.

4. Genc S, Koroglu TF, Genc K. Erythropoietin as a novel neuroprotectant. Restor Neurol Neurosci 2004;22(2):105–19.

5. Chong ZZ, Kang JQ, Maiese K. Angiogenesis and plasticity: role of erythropoietin in vascular systems. J Hematother Stem Cell Res 2002;11(6):863 71.

6. Sato T, Maekawa T, Watanabe S, et al. Erythroid progenitors differentiate and mature in response to endogenous erythropoietin. J Clin Invest 2000; 106(2):263 70.

7. Jelkmann W, Wagner K. Beneficial and ominous aspects of the pleiotropic action of erythropoietin. Ann Hematol 2004;83(11):673–86.

8. Anagnostou A, Lee ES, Kessimian N, et al. Erythropoietin has a mitogenic and positive chemotactic effect on endothelial cells. Proc Natl Acad Sci U S A 1990; 87(15):5978–82.

9. Maiese K, Li F, Chong ZZ. New avenues of exploration for erythropoietin. JAMA 2005;293(1):90–5.

10. Anagnostou A, Liu Z, Steiner M, et al. Erythropoietin receptor mRNA expression in human endothelial cells. Proc Natl Acad Sci U S A 1994;91(9):3974–8.

11. Morishita E, Narita H, Nishida M, et al. Anti-erythropoietin receptor monoclonal antibody: epitope mapping, quantification of the soluble receptor, and detection of the solubilized transmembrane receptor and the receptor-expressing cells. Blood 1996;88(2):465–71.

12. Chin K, Yu X, Beleslin-Cokic B, et al. Production and processing of erythropoietin receptor transcripts in brain. Brain Res Mol Brain Res 2000;81(1–2):29–42.

13. Liu C, Shen K, Liu Z, et al. Regulated human erythropoietin receptor expression in mouse brain. J Biol Chem 1997;272(51):32395–400.

14. Chong ZZ, Kang JQ, Maiese K. Hematopoietic factor erythropoietin fosters neuroprotection through novel signal transduction cascades. J Cereb Blood Flow Metab 2002;22(5):503–14.

15. Dzietko M, Felderhoff-Mueser U, Sifringer M, et al. Erythropoietin protects the developing brain against N-methyl-D-aspartate receptor antagonist neurotoxicity. Neurobiol Dis 2004;15(2):177–87.

16. Henry DH, Bowers P, Romano MT, et al. Epoetin alfa: clinical evolution of a pleiotropic cytokine. Arch Intern Med 2004;164(3):262–76.

17. Maiese K, Li F, Chong ZZ. Erythropoietin in the brain: can the promise to protect be fulfilled? Trends Pharmacol Sci 2004;25(11):577–83.

18. Constantinescu SN, Ghaffari S, Lodish HF. The erythropoietin receptor: structure, activation and intracellular signal transduction. Trends Endocrinol Metab 1999;10(1):18–23.

19. Brines M, Cerami A. Emerging biological roles for erythropoietin in the nervous system. Nat Rev Neurosci 2005;6(6):484–94.

20. Hewitson KS, McNeill LA, Schofield CJ. Modulating the hypoxia-inducible factor signaling pathway: applications from cardiovascular disease to cancer. Curr Pharm Des 2004;10(8):821–33.

21. Rankin EB, Biju MP, Liu Q, et al. Hypoxia-inducible factor-2 (HIF-2) regulates hepatic erythropoietin in vivo. J Clin Invest 2007;117(4):1068–77.

22. Tramontano AF, Muniyappa R, Black AD, et al. Erythropoietin protects cardiac myocytes from hypoxia-induced apoptosis through an Akt-dependent pathway. Biochem Biophys Res Commun 2003; 308(4):990–4.

23. Ratajczak J, Majka M, Kijowski J, et al. Biological significance of MAPK, AKT and JAK-STAT protein activation by various erythropoietic factors in normal human early erythroid cells. Br J Haematol 2001; 115(1):195–204.

24. Kawakami M, Sekiguchi M, Sato K, et al. Erythropoietin receptor-mediated inhibition of exocytotic glutamate release confers neuroprotection during chemical ischemia. J Biol Chem 2001;276(42):39469–75.

25. Hanlon PR, Fu P, Wright GL, et al. Mechanisms of erythropoietin-mediated cardioprotection during ischemia-reperfusion injury: role of protein kinase C and phosphatidylinositol 3-kinase signaling. FASEB J 2005;19(10):1323 5.

26. Bullard AJ, Govewalla P, Yellon DM. Erythropoietin protects the myocardium against reperfusion injury in vitro and in vivo. Basic Res Cardiol 2005;100(5): 397–403.

27. Chong ZZ, Li F, Maiese K. Activating Akt and the brain's resources to drive cellular survival and prevent inflammatory injury. Histol Histopathol 2005;20(1):299–315.

28. Chong ZZ, Kang JQ, Maiese K. Erythropoietin is a novel vascular protectant through activation of Akt1 and mitochondrial modulation of cysteine proteases. Circulation 2002;106(23):2973–9.

29. Chong ZZ, Kang JQ, Maiese K. Apaf-1, Bcl-xL, cytochrome c, and caspase-9 form the critical elements

for cerebral vascular protection by erythropoietin. J Cereb Blood Flow Metab 2003;23(3):320–30.

30. Kang JQ, Chong ZZ, Maiese K. Critical role for Akt1 in the modulation of apoptotic phosphatidylserine exposure and microglial activation. Mol Pharmacol 2003;64(3):557–69.

31. Kang PM, Izumo S. Apoptosis in heart: basic mechanisms and implications in cardiovascular diseases. Trends Mol Med 2003;9(4):177–82.

32. Wick A, Wick W, Waltenberger J, et al. Neuroprotection by hypoxic preconditioning requires sequential activation of vascular endothelial growth factor receptor and Akt. J Neurosci 2002;22(15):6401–7.

33. Lin CS, Lim SK, D'Agati V, et al. Differential effects of an erythropoietin receptor gene disruption on primitive and definitive erythropoiesis. Genes Dev 1996; 10(2):154–64.

34. Kieran MW, Perkins AC, Orkin SH, et al. Thrombopoietin rescues in vitro erythroid colony formation from mouse embryos lacking the erythropoietin receptor. Proc Natl Acad Sci U S A 1996;93(17): 9126–31.

35. Wu H, Liu X, Jaenisch R, et al. Generation of committed erythroid BFU-E and CFU-E progenitors does not require erythropoietin or the erythropoietin receptor. Cell 1995;83(1):59–67.

36. Wu H, Lee SH, Gao J, et al. Inactivation of erythropoietin leads to defects in cardiac morphogenesis. Development 1999;126(16):3597–605.

37. Suzuki N, Ohneda O, Takahashi S, et al. Erythroid-specific expression of the erythropoietin receptor rescued its null mutant mice from lethality. Blood 2002;100(7):2279–88.

38. Tada H, Kagaya Y, Takeda M, et al. Endogenous erythropoietin system in non-hematopoietic lineage cells plays a protective role in myocardial ischemia/reperfusion. Cardiovasc Res 2006;71(3): 466–77.

39. Asaumi Y, Kagaya Y, Takeda M, et al. Protective role of endogenous erythropoietin system in nonhematopoietic cells against pressure overload-induced left ventricular dysfunction in mice. Circulation 2007; 115(15):2022–32.

40. Satoh K, Kagaya Y, Nakano M, et al. Important role of endogenous erythropoietin system in recruitment of endothelial progenitor cells in hypoxia-induced pulmonary hypertension in mice. Circulation 2006; 113(11):1442–50.

41. van Albada ME, du Marchie Sarvaas GJ, Koster J, et al. Effects of erythropoietin on advanced pulmonary vascular remodelling. Eur Respir J 2008; 31(1):126–34.

42. Vairano M, Dello Russo C, Pozzoli G, et al. Erythropoietin exerts anti-apoptotic effects on rat microglial cells in vitro. Eur J Neurosci 2002;16(4):584–92.

43. Campana WM, Myers RR. Exogenous erythropoietin protects against dorsal root ganglion apoptosis and

pain following peripheral nerve injury. Eur J Neurosci 2003;18(6):1497–506.

44. Vesey DA, Cheung C, Pat B, et al. Erythropoietin protects against ischaemic acute renal injury. Nephrol Dial Transplant 2004;19(2):348–55.

45. Sekiguchi N, Inoguchi T, Kobayashi K, et al. Effect of erythropoietin on endothelial cell apoptosis induced by high glucose. Diabetes Res Clin Pract 2004; 66(Suppl 1):S103–7.

46. Yatsiv I, Grigoriadis N, Simeonidou C, et al. Erythropoietin is neuroprotective, improves functional recovery, and reduces neuronal apoptosis and inflammation in a rodent model of experimental closed head injury. FASEB J 2005;19(12):1701–3.

47. Smith KJ, Bleyer AJ, Little WC, et al. The cardiovascular effects of erythropoietin. Cardiovasc Res 2003; 59(3):538–48.

48. Lipsic E, van der Meer P, Henning RH, et al. Timing of erythropoietin treatment for cardioprotection in ischemia/reperfusion. J Cardiovasc Pharmacol 2004;44(4):473–9.

49. Parsa CJ, Matsumoto A, Kim J, et al. A novel protective effect of erythropoietin in the infarcted heart. J Clin Invest 2003;112(7):999–1007.

50. Cai Z, Semenza GL. Phosphatidylinositol-3-kinase signaling is required for erythropoietin-mediated acute protection against myocardial ischemia/reperfusion injury. Circulation 2004;109(17):2050–3.

51. Lipsic E, Schoemaker RG, van der Meer P, et al. Protective effects of erythropoietin in cardiac ischemia: from bench to bedside. J Am Coll Cardiol 2006;48(11):2161–7.

52. Calvillo L, Latini R, Kajstura J, et al. Recombinant human erythropoietin protects the myocardium from ischemia-reperfusion injury and promotes beneficial remodeling. Proc Natl Acad Sci U S A 2003;100(8):4802–6.

53. Parsa CJ, Kim J, Riel RU, et al. Cardioprotective effects of erythropoietin in the reperfused ischemic heart: a potential role for cardiac fibroblasts. J Biol Chem 2004;279(20):20655–62.

54. Hirata A, Minamino T, Asanuma H, et al. Erythropoietin enhances neovascularization of ischemic myocardium and improves left ventricular dysfunction after myocardial infarction in dogs. J Am Coll Cardiol 2006;48(1):176–84.

55. Gao E, Boucher M, Chuprun JK, et al. Darbepoetin alfa, a long-acting erythropoietin analog, offers novel and delayed cardioprotection for the ischemic heart. Am J Physiol Heart Circ Physiol 2007;293(1):H60–8.

56. van der Meer P, Lipsic E, Henning RH, et al. Erythropoietin improves left ventricular function and coronary flow in an experimental model of ischemia-reperfusion injury. Eur J Heart Fail 2004;6(7):853–9.

57. Fiordaliso F, Chimenti S, Staszewsky L, et al. A non-erythropoietic derivative of erythropoietin protects

the myocardium from ischemia-reperfusion injury. Proc Natl Acad Sci U S A 2005;102(6):2046–51.

58. de Boer RA, van Veldhuisen DJ, van der Wijk J, et al. Additional use of immunostaining for active caspase 3 and cleaved actin and PARP fragments to detect apoptosis in patients with chronic heart failure. J Card Fail 2000;6(4):330–7.

59. de Boer RA, Pinto YM, van Veldhuisen DJ. The imbalance between oxygen demand and supply as a potential mechanism in the pathophysiology of heart failure: the role of microvascular growth and abnormalities. Microcirculation 2003;10(2): 113–26.

60. Rodriguez M, Lucchesi BR, Schaper J. Apoptosis in myocardial infarction. Ann Med 2002;34(6):470–9.

61. Yellon DM, Hausenloy DJ. Myocardial reperfusion injury. N Engl J Med 2007;357(11):1121–35.

62. Ehrenreich H, Hasselblatt M, Dembowski C, et al. Erythropoietin therapy for acute stroke is both safe and beneficial. Mol Med 2002;8(8):495–505.

63. Ehrenreich H, Hinze-Selch D, Stawicki S, et al. Improvement of cognitive functions in chronic schizophrenic patients by recombinant human erythropoietin. Mol Psychiatry 2007;12(2):206–20.

64. Cariou A, Claessens YE, Pene F, et al. Early high-dose erythropoietin therapy and hypothermia after out-of-hospital cardiac arrest: a matched control study. Resuscitation 2008;76(3):397–404.

65. Ehrenreich H, Weissenborn K, Prange H, et al. Recombinant human erythropoietin in the treatment of acute ischemic stroke. Stroke 2009;40(12): e647–56.

66. Lipsic E, van der Meer P, Voors AA, et al. A single bolus of a long-acting erythropoietin analogue darbepoetin alfa in patients with acute myocardial infarction: a randomized feasibility and safety study. Cardiovasc Drugs Ther 2006;20(2):135–41.

67. Liem A, van de Woestijne AP, Bruijns E, et al. Effect of EPO administration on myocardial infarct size in patients with non-STE acute coronary syndromes: results from a pilot study. Int J Cardiol 2009;131(2): 285–7.

68. Cleland JG, Coletta AP, Clark AL, et al. Clinical trials update from the American College of Cardiology 2009: ADMIRE-HF, PRIMA, STICH, REVERSE, IRIS, partial ventricular support, FIX-HF-5, vagal stimulation, REVIVAL-3, pre-RELAX-AHF, ACTIVE-A, HF-ACTION, JUPITER, AURORA, and OMEGA. Eur J Heart Fail 2009;11(6):622–30.

69. Binbrek AS, Rao NS, Al Khaja N, et al. Erythropoietin to augment myocardial salvage induced by coronary thrombolysis in patients with ST segment elevation acute myocardial infarction. Am J Cardiol 2009; 104(8):1035–40.

70. Tang YD, Hasan F, Giordano FJ, et al. Effects of recombinant human erythropoietin on platelet activation in acute myocardial infarction: results of a double-blind, placebo-controlled, randomized trial. Am Heart J 2009;158(6):941–7.

71. Belonje AM, Voors AA, van Gilst WH, et al. Effects of erythropoietin after an acute myocardial infarction: rationale and study design of a prospective, randomized, clinical trial (HEBE III). Am Heart J 2008;155(5):817–22.

72. Reduction of infarct expansion and ventricular remodeling with erythropoietin after large myocardial infarction (REVEAL). 2009. Available at: http://www.clinicaltrials.gov. Accessed December 16, 2009.

73. Namiuchi S, Kagaya Y, Ohta J, et al. High serum erythropoietin level is associated with smaller infarct size in patients with acute myocardial infarction who undergo successful primary percutaneous coronary intervention. J Am Coll Cardiol 2005;45(9):1406–12.

74. Drueke TB, Locatelli F, Clyne N, et al. Normalization of hemoglobin level in patients with chronic kidney disease and anemia. N Engl J Med 2006;355(20): 2071–84.

75. Singh AK, Szczech L, Tang KL, et al. Correction of anemia with epoetin alfa in chronic kidney disease. N Engl J Med 2006;355(20):2085–98.

76. Lipsic E, Westenbrink BD, van der Meer P, et al. Low-dose erythropoietin improves cardiac function in experimental heart failure without increasing haematocrit. Eur J Heart Fail 2008;10(1):22–9.

77. Bahlmann FH, Song R, Boehm SM, et al. Low-dose therapy with the long-acting erythropoietin analogue darbepoetin alpha persistently activates endothelial Akt and attenuates progressive organ failure. Circulation 2004;110(8):1006–12.

78. Leist M, Ghezzi P, Grasso G, et al. Derivatives of erythropoietin that are tissue protective but not erythropoietic. Science 2004;305(5681):239–42.

Therapy with Erythropoiesis-Stimulating Agents and Renal and Nonrenal Outcomes

Anil K. Agarwal, MD[a], Ajay K. Singh, MB, FRCP(UK)[b],*

KEYWORDS

- Epoetin • Epogen • Erythropoiesis-stimulating agents
- CKD • ESRD

The use of erythropoiesis-stimulating agents (ESA) in the treatment of the anemia of heart failure or chronic kidney disease (CKD) is currently controversial.[1,2] A large number of observational studies have reported an association between the severity of anemia in patients with CKD and heart failure (HF) and outcomes such as mortality and hospitalization risk.[3–10] These studies are reviewed extensively elsewhere. In CKD patients on dialysis and those not on dialysis, higher hemoglobin concentrations are associated with a lower risk of mortality, cardiovascular complications, and hospitalization. In patients with heart failure, a study by McClellan and colleagues[6] examining a retrospective cohort of 655 Medicare patients admitted to community hospitals for heart failure reported a 2.4% decrease in 1-year risk of death per 1% increase in hematocrit after adjustment for age, sex, race, kidney function, and cardiovascular comorbidities (**Table 1**). Other studies have found an association between anemia and the risk of hospitalization.[7–10] On the other hand, there has been a paucity of evidence from randomized controlled studies to indicate that correction of

anemia is associated with benefit. In patients with CKD, several randomized controlled trials (RCTs) indicate that the use of ESA in correcting anemia is associated with increased risk.[11–14] Consequently, we are left with a conundrum: although anemia is common in HF and CKD and observational studies indicate benefit with higher hemoglobin concentrations, treatment with ESA used to target a higher hemoglobin is associated with increased risk of adverse outcomes. For the clinician, the treatment questions are simple: should we be treating CKD and/or HF anemia with an ESA? If so, what level of hemoglobin should be targeted? This article examines the observational data and the recent information from randomized trials that point to increased risk in CKD and HF settings, and whether these disparate results can be explained by exposure to ESAs in this setting.

RENAL OUTCOMES IN ANEMIA

Anemia is a common complication of CKD and progresses with deterioration of kidney function.[15]

Disclosures: Dr Agarwal has received honoraria from Amgen and is an investigator in TREAT. He has received research support from Amgen, Fibrogen, and AMAG. Dr Singh was Principal Investigator of the CHOIR study and a member of the Executive Committee for the TREAT study. He reports receiving consulting income from Amgen, Johnson & Johnson, Fibrogen, and Watson. He reports receiving grant support from Amgen, Johnson & Johnson and Watson.
[a] Division of Nephrology, The Ohio State University, 395 West 12th Avenue, Ground Floor, Columbus, OH 43210, USA
[b] Renal Division, Brigham and Women's Hospital, Harvard Medical School, 75 Francis Street, Boston, MA 02115, USA
* Corresponding author.
E-mail address: asingh@rics.bwh.harvard.edu

Heart Failure Clin 6 (2010) 323–332
doi:10.1016/j.hfc.2010.03.006
1551-7136/10/$ – see front matter © 2010 Elsevier Inc. All rights reserved.

Table 1
In heart failure, higher hematocrit is associated with lower risk of death

Hematocrit (%)	Percent of Patients	1-Year Mortality (%)	Odds Ratio
>40	30.3	31.3	1.0
36–39	22.9	33.8	1.08
30–35	33.2	36.7	1.17
<30	13.6	50.0	1.60

Data from McClellan WM, Flanders WD, Langston RD, et al. Anemia and renal insufficiency are independent risk factors for death among patients with congestive heart failure admitted to community hospitals: a population-based study. J Am Soc Nephrol 2002;13(7):1928–36.

At the onset of dialysis, almost three-quarters of all patients have anemia. The primary cause of anemia of CKD is an actual or relative deficiency of erythropoietin (EPO) as a result of decreased production from diseased kidney.

The relationship of anemia to renal disease progression has been examined in multiple observational and prospective studies.[16–22] Evidence from observational studies suggests that anemia is an independent predictor of adverse outcomes in CKD.[16–22] In these studies, a lower hemoglobin level has been linked as an independent predictor for the development of end-stage renal disease (ESRD) in a linear fashion.[23–25]

Data from early animal studies demonstrated faster decline in renal function with treatment of anemia with recombinant EPO.[26,27] The mechanism of this decline in animals was unclear, although an increase in blood pressure and an increase in blood viscosity with the rapid increase in hematocrit have been invoked to explain the accelerated glomerular injury. On the other hand, observational data from several human studies do not support this conclusion.[28–30] For example, Jungers and colleagues[28] reported that anemia treatment retards the decline in estimated glomerular filtration rate (GFR) from −0.36 mL/min/mo in an ESA-untreated group to −0.26 mL/min/mo with ESA treatment. In a retrospective observational study of older patients with renal insufficiency, treatment with ESA slowed the decline in eGFR (by Cockcroft Gault formula) from −0.094 dL/mg/y to −0.057 dL/mg/y.[29] An increase in hematocrit from 26.9% to 33.1% led to a slower slope of loss of renal function in another study.[30]

Smaller prospective studies have also reported that ESA treatment retards the slope of progression of kidney dysfunction in advanced kidney disease. In a study by Roth and colleagues,[31] patients with severe CKD (mean eGFR 10 mL/min) and a baseline mean hematocrit of 26.8%, experienced a decline in GFR of −0.13 mL/min/mo with ESA treatment compared with −0.39/min/mo in the control group, reflecting a 3 times greater slowing in the rate of decline in GFR with ESA treatment. In another prospective study by Kuriyama and colleagues,[32] 2 groups of patients with CKD with serum creatinine level of 2 to 4 mg/dL with anemia (hematocrit <30) were randomized to ESA or no ESA, and were compared with a control group of patients with hematocrit greater than 30. Blood pressure was comparably controlled and other renoprotective measures were taken in both groups. Renal survival for a follow-up period of 18 to 36 months was significantly better in the nonanemic controls and those treated with ESA than in those with lower hematocrit and no ESA therapy. The improvement in renal survival was especially prominent in those without noninsulin-dependent diabetes mellitus. Another randomized, prospective, controlled study of nondiabetic patients with serum creatinine level between 2 and 6 mg/dL was stratified according to hemoglobin level.[33] Those with hemoglobin between 9 and 11.6 g/dL were treated immediately (early group), whereas those in the deferred group were only treated with erythropoietin-stimulating protein when hemoglobin decreased to less than 9 g/dL. The median follow-up was 22.5 months, with achieved hemoglobin level of 12.9 g/dL in the early arm and 10.3 g/dL in the deferred arm. There was a 60% reduction in death or renal replacement in patients in the early treatment arm. Collectively, these studies suggested that early treatment of anemia with ESA retards the progression of renal disease, and the outcomes may be especially significant in diabetic kidney disease. (The difference between diabetic and nondiabetic disease may be the result of earlier occurrence of anemia in patients with diabetic kidney disease). However, all these trials are limited by their small sample size and problems in design.

Larger randomized studies have been conducted to test the hypothesis of whether ESA treatment in CKD anemia slows down progression of renal disease.[12–14] **Table 2** summarizes their design. The conclusion from these studies does not support a beneficial effect of anemia correction with ESA on renal progression. The Cardiovascular Risk reduction by Early Anemia Treatment with Epoetin beta (CREATE) study, an open-label randomized multicenter trial conducted in Europe, evaluated the effect of complete versus partial correction of anemia on cardiovascular disease (CVD) risk reduction in 600 patients with CKD.[12] Achieved hemoglobin was 13.49 g/dL in the high-hemoglobin target group versus 11.6 g/dL in the standard target group. At 4-year follow-up there was no statistical difference in CVD events or left ventricular mass index between the groups. A prespecified secondary analysis showed a higher risk of developing ESRD requiring dialysis in patients randomized to the higher hemoglobin concentration. In the higher hemoglobin group, 127 patients developed ESRD compared with 111 patients in the low hemoglobin group. There was a statistically significant difference in the time to initiation of dialysis. The higher hemoglobin group had a shorter time to dialysis compared with the lower hemoglobin group (P = .03) The Correction of Hemoglobin and Outcomes in Renal Insufficiency (CHOIR) study, an open-label, prospective, randomized trial of EPO in 1432 patients with CKD anemia, compared the effect of increasing the hemoglobin concentration to high (13.5 g/dL) versus low (11.3 g/dL) levels.[13] There were 125 composite events (death, myocardial infarction, congestive heart failure [CHF], hospitalization, and stroke) among the patients in the higher hemoglobin group and 97 events among those in the low hemoglobin group (hazard ratio [HR]of 1.337, P = .03). In CHOIR there was a strong trend to a higher rate of dialysis requiring renal replacement therapy in the higher hemoglobin group (155 patients or 21.7% in the higher hemoglobin arm versus 134 patients or 18.7% in the lower hemoglobin arm (HR 1.186, 95% confidence interval [CI] 0.941, 1.495)). In patients requiring hospitalization for renal replacement therapy, the risk was greater in patients randomized to the higher hemoglobin arm (13.8% vs 11.3) (HR 1.253, 95% CI 0.934, 1.680). The Trial to Reduce Cardiovascular Events with Aranesp Therapy (TREAT) study[14] was a large, multinational, randomized controlled double-blind trial comprising 4038 subjects. The patients were treated with darbepoetin or placebo, with a target hemoglobin level of 13 g/dL. Rescue darbepoetin treatment was given to those with hemoglobin level less than 9 g/dL in the placebo arm. Six hundred and thirty-two patients were assigned to darbepoetin-alfa and 602 patients were assigned to placebo (HR for darbepoetin vs placebo 1.05;

Table 2
Comparison of the design of CREATE, CHOIR, and TREAT

	CREATE		CHOIR	TREAT
Design	Randomized, open-label		Randomized, open-label	Randomized, double-blind, controlled
Sponsor/agent	Roche/Neorecormon (epoetin-beta)		J&J/Procrit (epoetin-alfa)	Amgen/Aranesp (darbepoetin-alfa)
Design	Open-label		Open-label	Double-blind
Dosing	2,000 QW		Initiate 10,000 QW When stable go to Q2W	0.75 µg/kg/Q2W Double dose when stable and go to QM
Dosing frequency	De novo to QW		De novo to QW to Q2W	De novo to Q2W to QM
Hb target(s), g/L	Arm 1	13.0–15.0	13.5	13.0
	Arm 2	10.5–11.5*	11.3	Placebo (rescue for Hb <9.0)
Regions	Global		United States	Global
Inclusion				
Hb (g/L)	11.0–12.5		<11.0	≤11.0
eGFR/CrCl	15–35		15–50	20–60
Diabetes	No (~25%)		No (48.5%)	Yes (100%)

Abbreviations: QM, every month; Q2W, every 2 weeks; QW, every week.

P = .41). TREAT was neutral for its primary composite end points: death or a cardiovascular event or death or ESRD. Death or ESRD occurred in 652 patients in the darbepoetin-alfa group (32.4%) and in 618 patients in the placebo group (30.5%) (HR for darbepoetin-alfa vs placebo 1.06; 95% CI 0.95–1.19; P = .29). ESRD occurred in 338 patients in the darbepoetin-alfa group (16.8%) and in 330 patients assigned to placebo (16.3%) (HR 1.02; 95% CI 0.87–1.18; P = .83). Thus, in CREATE, CHOIR, and TREAT there was no retardation of renal progression; on the contrary, there was increased risk (CREATE) or no benefit (CHOIR, TREAT) for renal outcomes with anemia correction.

CARDIOVASCULAR OUTCOMES WITH ESA TREATMENT IN HF

Anemia has not been previously recognized as a risk factor for HF in the guidelines for HF.[34] However, anemia is common in HF (~20%–30% of patients) and seems to be mulifactorial (**Table 3**). It remains unclear whether treatment of anemia with ESA improves outcomes in patients with HF. The potential benefits for treating anemia in HF patients are

- Improved oxygen delivery
- Attenuate adverse cardiac remodeling
- Improved exercise tolerance
- Improved health-related quality of life
- Reduce ischemia and ischemic myocardial damage through inhibiting myocardial apoptosis.

The effect of anemia correction in HF has been studied in several small noncontrolled and controlled trials. In a small (n = 26) noncontrolled study, there was significant clinical improvement by increasing hemoglobin levels from 10 g to 12 g using EPO and iron therapy.[35] Similar results were obtained in a small controlled study.[36,37]

Continued evidence for a beneficial effect of ESA has been accumulating in recent RCTs. A phase II trial of ESA in patients with HF (n = 475) showed improvement in hemoglobin level and in HF symptoms, with improved exercise capacity.[38] A small (n = 41) multicenter, randomized, placebo-controlled, double-blind study of ESA with or without oral iron aimed at a target hemoglobin level of 10 to 15 g.[39] There was significant improvement in self-reported global assessment of change, but the changes in oxygen consumption and exercise duration were not significant. A larger (n = 165) multicenter, double-blind, placebo-controlled study of darbepoetin treatment with a target hemoglobin level of 14 g also failed to improve New York Heart Association (NYHA) class with significant improvement in Kansas City Cardiomyopathy symptom score.[40] There were 6 deaths in the ESA group, compared with none in the placebo-controlled group. STAMINA-HeFT, another large (n = 319) randomized, placebo-controlled trial of darbepoetin-alfa to increase hemoglobin level to 14 g in HF patients did not demonstrate significant improvement in exercise duration, quality of life, or NYHA functional class with treatment of anemia to a high target.[41]

In a recent single-center retrospective study of patients with HF (n = 6159), anemia was associated with advanced NYHA functional class, worse renal function, old age, diabetes mellitus, and neurohormonal activation.[45] In this study,

Table 3
Potential causes of anemia in HF

Reduced cardiac output	Reduced renal perfusion, leading to impaired renal function, and decreased erythropoietin production
	Reduced bone marrow perfusion leading to impaired function and anemia
Inflammation	Induction of a proinflammatory state with high levels of tumor necrosis factor and other inflammatory cytokines; increased hepcidin levels, reduced bone marrow responsiveness
Iron deficiency	Increased hepcidin levels result in reduced absorption and mobilization of iron
Angiotensin-converting enzyme (ACE) inhibitors	Down-regulation of erythropoietin synthesis by ACE inhibitors
Dilutional	Plasma volume expansion

new-onset anemia and persistent anemia were associated with significant risk of mortality (20% increase with each 1 g decrease in hemoglobin). Anemia at baseline improved in 43% of the patients and this transient decline in hemoglobin was not associated with increased risk of death. The Reduction of Events with Darbepoetin-alfa in Heart Failure (RED-HF) trial is an ongoing trial of darbepoetin-alfa in HF patients randomizing 3400 anemic patients with systolic HF in a double-blind fashion.

A recent meta-analysis of EPO treatment in patients with chronic HF considered 7 randomized controlled trials comparing ESA treatment with placebo.[46] Of the 650 patients enrolled, those treated with ESA (n = 363) had a lower risk of hospitalization compared with those treated with placebo (n = 287). A summary of the studies included is shown in **Table 4**. The treatment did not make any difference in mortality risk, occurrence of hypertension, or venous thrombosis. However, the quality of the studies included in this meta-analysis varied, making the effect on hospitalization more impressive.[47]

The RED-HF trial is a double-blind, randomized, placebo-controlled, parallel-group, multicenter study currently enrolling patients to examine the effect of ESA treatment on morbidity and mortality in patients with HF (NYHA class II–IV), ejection fraction less than or equal to 40%, and anemia. This study of 2600 patients with HF and hemoglobin levels between 9 and 12 g/dL will randomize patients to either placebo or darbepoetin-alfa with a target hemoglobin level of 13 g/dL.

CARDIOVASCULAR OUTCOMES IN CKD WITH ESA TREATMENT

In RCTs of patients with CKD, correction of anemia has not demonstrated improvement in cardiovascular end points. The Normal Hematocrit study found worse outcomes when dialysis patients with preexisting HF targeted to normal hemoglobin with epoetin-alfa.[11] The Normal Hematocrit study tested the hypothesis that the correction of anemia with epoetin-alfa (Epogen) in hemodialysis patients with clinical evidence of CHF or ischemic heart disease would result in improved outcomes. The primary end point was the length of time to death or a first nonfatal myocardial infarction. The study was halted at the third interim analysis on the recommendation of the Data Safety Monitoring Board. At 29 months, there were 183 deaths and 19 first nonfatal myocardial infarctions in the group with a normal hematocrit, and 150 deaths and 14 nonfatal myocardial infarctions in the low hematocrit group (RR 1.3; 95% CI 0.9–1.9). In the

Canada-Europe trial, subjects at high risk were excluded and the sample comprised of patients who had been recently initiated on dialysis and did not have known CVD.[48] There was no significant difference in change in the primary end point of left ventricular volume index (LVVI). RCTs evaluating nondialysis CKD patients (CREATE, CHOIR, and TREAT) are summarized in **Table 2**. In all 3 studies, no improvement with anemia correction in either a composite cardiovascular end point or the cardiovascular components of the composite end point was observed. In CHOIR the primary end point was a composite of death, myocardial infarction, CHF, hospitalization, and stroke. One hundred and twenty-five events occurred among the high-hemoglobin group and 97 events among the low hemoglobin group (HR 1.34; P = .03). The higher rate of composite events was explained largely by a higher rate of death (48% higher risk, P = .07) or CHF hospitalization (41%, P = .07). In CREATE, complete correction was not associated with a higher rate of the first cardiovascular event (HR 0.78; P = .20). TREAT was neutral for the primary composite of death or a cardiovascular event (HR for darbepoetin vs placebo 1.05; P = .41), but there was a significantly higher rate of strokes in patients treated with darbepoetin. Fatal or nonfatal strokes occurred in 101 patients assigned to darbepoetin and 53 patients assigned to placebo (HR 1.92; P<.001). Synthesizing data from the 4 large RCTs, In Normal Hematocrit, the point estimate of risk in the direction of harm was 30%; in CREATE, the risk in the direction of harm was 22% (95% CIs of 0.53 and 1.14); in CHOIR 34% (95% CI 1.03 and 1.74); and in TREAT 5% (95% CI 0.94–1.17), respectively. Thus, evidence for improvement in cardiovascular end points with treatment of anemia with ESA is lacking in patients with CKD.

IS EXPOSURE TO ESAS THE EXPLANATION FOR INCREASED RISK IN STUDIES CORRECTING ANEMIA IN CKD?

Observational studies suggest lower risk with higher hemoglobin concentrations,[3–5] whereas RCTs indicate higher risk associated with targeting a higher hemoglobin with ESA.[11–14] How can these disparate conclusions be reconciled? Is targeting and achieving a higher hemoglobin associated with increased risk? If so, then one would have to concede that the observational studies are hopelessly confounded. On the other hand, if the act of targeting a higher hemoglobin with higher doses of ESA but not the actual achieving of the higher hemoglobin was the reason for the increased risk, then normalizing the hemoglobin

Table 4
Summary of the studies included

First Author and Publication Date	Follow-up	n	Patients	Major Exclusion Criteria	End Points	ESP	Target Hb or Ht	Study Design	Study Quality
Parissis, 2008[42]	3 months	32	NYHA II–III LVEF <40% Hb <12.5 g/dL	sCr >2.5 mg/dL	Exercise capacity Echocardiographic LV and RV evaluation	Darbepoetin-alfa	14.0 g/dL	Randomized, single-blind, placebo-controlled, single-center study	Fair
Ghali et al,[41] 2008	1 year	319	NYHA II–IV LVEF <40% Hb <12.5 g/dL	sCr >3.0 mg/dL	Change in exercise time NYHA class, mortality HF hospitalization	Darbepoetin-alfa	14.0 g/dL	Randomized, double-blind, placebo-controlled, multicenter study	Fair
Van Veldhuisen,[43] 2007	26 weeks	165	Symptomatic HF LVEF <40% Hb 9.0–12.5 g/dL	sCr >3.0 mg/dL	Hb increase, 6-minute walk distance, safety	Darbepoetin-alfa	14.0 g/dL	Randomized, double-blind, placebo-controlled, multicenter study	Fair
Ponikowski et al,[39] 2007	26 weeks	41	Symptomatic CHF LVEF <40% Hb 9–12 g/dL	Blood transfusion or ESP within 12 weeks sCr >3.0 mg/dL	Exercise tolerance and duration, NYHA, BNP, hospitalization	Darbepoetin-alfa	Hb 13.0–15.0 g/dL	Randomized, double-blind, placebo-controlled, multicenter study	Fair
Mancini et al,[37] 2003	3 months	23	NYHA III/IV Ht <35%,	Non-ambulatory patients, continuous inotropic agents, iron deficiency anemia sCr >2.5 mg/dL	Exercise performance	Erythropoietin alfa	Ht >45%	Randomized, single-blind, placebo-controlled, single-center study	Fair
Palazzuoli, 2006[44]	3 months	38	NYHA III/IV Hb <11 g/dL	Secondary causes of anemia, isolated diastolic HF, <12 weeks MI sCr >5.0 mg/dL	NYHA class, exercise capacity, renal function, O2 use, BNP	Erythropoietin beta	Hb 11.5–12.0 g/dL	Randomized, double-blind, placebo-controlled, single-center study	Fair
Silverberg et al,[36] 2001	8.2 months	32	LVEF <40% Hb 10–11.5 g/dL	Secondary causes of anemia	Days of hospitalization	Erythropoietin	12.5 g/dL	Randomized, open-label, single-center study	Fair

Abbreviations: BNP, B-type natriuretic protein; CHF, chronic heart failure; ESP, erythropoietin-stimulating protein; Ht, hematocrit; LV, left ventricular; LVEF, left ventricular ejection fraction; MI, myocardial infarction; NYHA, New York Heart Association; RV, right ventricular; sCr, serum creatinine.

From van der Meer P, Groenveld HF, Januzzi JL Jr, et al. Erythropoietin treatment in patients with chronic heart failure: a meta-analysis. Heart 2009;95:1309–14; with permission.

per se would be safe as long as low doses or physiologic administration of ESA were pursued.

Several studies representing observational analyses or post hoc or planned secondary analyses of RCTs have examined the relationship between erythropoietin exposure and adverse risk in treating anemia in the CKD population.[49-55] Observational analyses have generated conflicting results. Some studies have reported a strong independent association between exposure to high doses of ESA and adverse outcome, whereas others have been unsupportive. One common theme has emerged however. In secondary analysis of the RCTs, higher achieved hemoglobin concentration is associated with better outcome, whereas lower achieved hemoglobin is associated with worse outcome. Observational analyses and the RCTs are therefore compatible with respect to the relationship between achieved hemoglobin and outcome. Thus, increased attention is now being directed at the issue of targeting a higher hemoglobin. Targeting a higher hemoglobin requires higher doses of ESA, therefore a logical inference has been that exposure to ESA itself perhaps under certain circumstances, such as in the context of inflammation or in patients with higher hemoglobin, accounts for increased risk. Several studies have examined this hypothesis and at least so far the results are inconsistent.

Zhang and colleagues[49] retrospectively studied a cohort of 94,569 prevalent hemodialysis patients from 2000 and 2001. A Cox proportional hazard regression analysis with adjustment for baseline variables was performed to examine the dose-response relationship between erythropoietin and all-cause mortality. For every hematocrit strata studied, patients administered higher doses of erythropoietin had significantly lower hematocrit values and greater mortality. With the cubic spline function, a significant nonlinear relationship between increased erythropoietin dose and mortality was found regardless of hematocrit value ($P = .0001$), with the steepest increase in relative risk for death found after the 75th dose percentile.

Streja and colleagues[52] studied a cohort of 40,787 maintenance hemodialysis patients and examined predictors of 3-year survival. A higher hemoglobin concentration greater than 13 g/dL was associated with greater mortality (case-mix-adjusted death relative risk of 1.21, 95% CI 1.02-1.44, $P = .03$) in the presence of thrombocytosis (platelet count >300,000/L) but not in the absence of thrombocytosis. There was an association with erythropoietin exposure; however, this was at very high erythropoietin doses of 20,000 units/wk and mortality over 3 years (relative risk of death 1.59, 95% CI 1.54-1.65, $P = .001$).

Bradbury and colleagues[53] have explored a Fresenius North America cohort of 22,955 patients. The relationship among erythropoietin dose, hemoglobin concentration, and baseline patient characteristics was also evaluated using Cox proportional hazard models and time-dependent models fitted with time-varying log erythropoietin and hemoglobin concentrations. In the unadjusted model, the investigators observed an increased mortality risk with an increasing erythropoietin dose (HR of 1.31 per log unit increase, 95% CI 1.26-1.36). However, adjustment for baseline patient characteristics resulted in attenuation in the mortality risk estimate (HR 1.21, 95% CI 1.15-1.28). In the lagged time-dependent analyses, the risk estimates further attenuated with estimates that ranged from HR of 0.93 (95% CI 0.92-0.95) to HR of 1.01 (95% CI 0.99-1.03) for the 1- and 2-month lagged models, respectively. These data suggested a potential association between erythropoietin exposure and mortality but the mortality risk estimate was highly sensitive to the analytical method used.

In the study by Zhang and colleagues,[54] inverse probability weighting was used to adjust for time-dependent confounding by indication. A sample of 18,454 patients from the United States Renal Data System (USRDS) database was used for the analysis. The association between cumulative average erythropoietin dosage and survival was explored. Zhang and colleagues reported that survival was similar for the 3 hypothetical erythropoietin treatment regimens selected: low dosage 15,000 units/wk, medium dosage 30,000 units/wk, and high dosage 45,000 units/wk of epoetin-alfa.

To further examine the relationship among erythropoietin dose, patient comorbidities, and outcome, Szczech and colleagues[55] performed a secondary analysis of the CHOIR study. An analytical approach called landmark analysis was applied to handle the problem of confounding. In unadjusted analyses, inability to achieve target hemoglobin concentrations and requirement of high-dose erythropoietin were significantly associated with an increased hazard of the primary end point ($P = .05$ and .003, respectively). In adjusted models, the increased hazard associated with randomization to the high-hemoglobin arm from the primary trial was no longer significant ($P = .49$), whereas high-dose erythropoietin was associated with a 57% increased hazard of the primary end point (HR 1.57, CI 1.04-2.36, $P = .03$). Hence, this study was compatible with the results of the other observational studies in suggesting that erythropoietin dose rather than the hemoglobin level is associated with adverse outcome.

Collectively, the data from observational analysis and secondary analysis of RCTs such as CHOIR, indicate that exposure to ESA at high doses might be important in explaining the higher risk with targeting a higher hemoglobin observed in the RCTs. However, the results were hypothesis testing and did not prove causality because one cannot totally exclude the possibility of confounding particularly from unmeasured confounding (residual confounding) or the influencing of dose targeting bias.

SUMMARY

The effect of ESAs on renal and cardiovascular outcomes in patients with CKD and HF is uncertain. Observational data indicate a strong relationship between the severity of anemia and poor outcome. On the other hand, RCTs on patients with CKD indicate that ESAs used in targeting a higher hemoglobin concentration result in increased risk. Because well-designed RCTs represent type A evidence, emphasizing RCTs rather than observational data is legitimate in assessing the safety of ESAs. Some have tried to separate HF from CKD in thinking about the risk of ESAs, arguing that patients with HF represent a different population and that smaller RCTs on HF (discussed in this review) have reported benefit. Whether exposure to high doses of ESA might explain the higher risk of mortality and cardiovascular complications in the RCTs in CKD and whether a similar phenomenon might be observed in other disease states, such as HF, remains unclear. Indeed, the mechanism of how ESAs might cause increased risk from a mechanistic perspective needs active investigation.

REFERENCES

1. Singh AK. Does TREAT give the boot to ESAs in the treatment of CKD anemia? J Am Soc Nephrol 2010; 21(1):2–6.
2. Singh AK. Resolved: targeting a higher hemoglobin is associated with greater risk in patients with CKD anemia: pro. J Am Soc Nephrol 2009;20:1436–41.
3. Collins AJ, Li S, St Peter W, et al. Death, hospitalization, and economic associations among incident hemodialysis patients with hematocrit values of 36 to 39%. J Am Soc Nephrol 2001;12(11):2465–73.
4. Regidor DL, Kopple JD, Kovesdy CP, et al. Associations between changes in hemoglobin and administered erythropoiesis-stimulating agent and survival in hemodialysis patients. J Am Soc Nephrol 2006; 17(4):1181–91.
5. Robinson BM, Joffe MM, Berns JS, et al. Anemia and mortality in hemodialysis patients: accounting for morbidity and treatment variables updated over time. Kidney Int 2005;68(5):2323–30.
6. McClellan WM, Flanders WD, Langston RD, et al. Anemia and renal insufficiency are independent risk factors for death among patients with congestive heart failure admitted to community hospitals: a population-based study. J Am Soc Nephrol 2002; 13(7):1928–36.
7. Alexander M, Baker L, Clark C, et al. Management of ventricular arrhythmias in diverse populations in California. Am Heart J 2002;144(3):431–9.
8. Polanczyk CA, Newton C, Dec GW, et al. Quality of care and hospital readmission in congestive heart failure: an explicit review process. J Card Fail 2001;7(4):289–98.
9. Felker GM, Gattis WA, Leimberger JD, et al. Usefulness of anemia as a predictor of death and rehospitalization in patients with decompensated heart failure. Am J Cardiol 2003;92(5):625–8.
10. Kosiborod M, Smith GL, Radford MJ, et al. The prognostic importance of anemia in patients with heart failure. Am J Med 2003;114(2):112–9.
11. Besarab A, Bolton WK, Browne JK, et al. The effects of normal as compared with low hematocrit values in patients with cardiac disease who are receiving hemodialysis and epoetin. N Engl J Med 1998;339: 584–90.
12. Drueke TB, Locatelli F, Clyne N, et al. Normalization of hemoglobin level in patients with chronic kidney disease and anemia. N Engl J Med 2006;355: 2071–84.
13. Singh AK, Szczech L, Tang KL, et al. Correction of anemia with epoetin alfa in chronic kidney disease. N Engl J Med 2006;355:2085–98.
14. Pfeffer MA, Burdmann EA, Chen CY, et al. A trial of darbepoetin alfa in type 2 diabetes and chronic kidney disease. N Engl J Med 2009;361(21):2019–32.
15. Radtke HW, Claussner A, Erbes PM, et al. Serum erythropoietin concentration in chronic renal failure: relationship to degree of anemia and excretory renal function. Blood 1978;54:877–84.
16. Breyer JA, Bain RP, Evans JK, et al. Predictors of the progression of renal insufficiency in patients with insulin dependent diabetes and overt diabetic nephropathy: the Collaborative Study Group. Kidney Int 1996;50:1651–8.
17. Hideki U, Ishimura E, Shoji T, et al. Factors affecting progression of renal failure in patients with type 2 diabetes. Diabetes Care 2003;26:1530–4.
18. Yokoyama H, Tomonaga O, Hirayama M, et al. Predictors of the progression of diabetic nephropathy and the beneficial effect of angiotensin-converting enzyme inhibitors in NIDDM patients. Diabetologia 1997;40:405–11.
19. Muirhead N. The rationale for early management of chronic renal insufficiency. Nephrol Dial Transplant 2001;16:51–6.

20. Klahr S. Prevention of progression of nephropathy. Nephrol Dial Transplant 1997;12:63–6.
21. van Ypersele de Strihou C. Should anaemia in subtypes of CRF patients be managed differently? Nephrol Dial Transplant 1999;14:37–45.
22. Peterson JC, Adler S, Burkart JM, et al. Blood pressure control, proteinuria, and the progression of renal disease: the modification of diet in renal disease study. Ann Intern Med 1995;123:754–62.
23. Iseki K, Ikemiya Y, Iseki C, et al. Haematocrit and the risk of developing end-stage renal disease. Nephrol Dial Transplant 2003;18:899–905.
24. Keane WF, Brenner BM, de Zeeuw D, et al. RENAAL study investigators. The risk of developing end stage renal disease in patients with type 2 diabetes and nephropathy: the RENAAL study. Kidney Int 2003;63:1499–507.
25. Cusick M, Chew EY, Hoogwerf B, et al. Early treatment diabetic retinopathy study research group. Risk factors for renal replacement therapy in the early treatment diabetic retinopathy study. Early treatment diabetic retinopathy study report no. 26. Kidney Int 2004;66:1173–9.
26. Garcia DL, Anderson S, Rennke HG, et al. Anemia lessens and its prevention worsens glomerular injury and hypertension in rats with reduced renal mass. Proc Natl Acad Sci U S A 1988;85:6142–6.
27. Myers BD, Deen WM, Robertson CR, et al. Dynamics of glomerular filtration in the rat. VIII. Effects of hematocrit. Circ Res 1975;36:425–35.
28. Jungers P, Choukroun G, Oualim Z, et al. Beneficial influence of recombinant human erythropoietin therapy on the rate of progression of chronic renal failure in predialysis patients. Nephrol Dial Transplant 2001;16:307–12.
29. Dean BB, Dylan M, Gano A Jr, et al. Erythropoiesis-stimulating protein therapy and the decline of renal function: a retrospective analysis of patients with chronic kidney disease. Curr Med Res Opin 2005;21:981–7.
30. Topolyai M, Kadomatsu S, Perera-Chong M. rhu-erythropoietin treatment of pre-ESRD patients slows the rate of progression of renal decline. BMC Nephrol 2003;4:3.
31. Roth D, Smith RD, Schulman G, et al. Effect of recombinant human erythropoietin on renal function in chronic renal failure predialysis patients. Am J Kidney Dis 1994;24:777–84.
32. Kuriyama S, Tomonari H, Yoshida H, et al. Reversal of anemia by erythropoietin therapy retards the progression of chronic renal failure, especially in nondiabetic patients. Nephron 1997;77:176–85.
33. Gouva C, Nikolopoulos P, Loannidis JP, et al. Treating anemia early in renal failure patients slows the decline of renal function: a randomized controlled trial. Kidney Int 2004;66:753–60.
34. Hunt SA, Baker DW, Chin MH, et al. ACC/AHA guidelines for the evaluation and management of chronic heart failure in the adult: executive summary: a report of the American College of Cardiology/American Heart Association Task Force on Practice Guidelines (Committee to Revise the 1995 Guidelines for the Evaluation and Management of Heart Failure). J Am Coll Cardiol 2001;38:2101–18.
35. Silverberg DS, Wexler D, Blum M, et al. The use of subcutaneous erythropoietin and intravenous iron for the treatment of the anemia of severe, resistant congestive HF improves cardiac and renal function and functional cardiac class, and markedly reduces hospitalizations. J Am Coll Cardiol 2000;35:1737–44.
36. Silverberg DS, Wexler D, Sheps D, et al. The effect of correction of mild anemia in severe, resistant congestive heart failure using subcutaneous erythropoietin and intravenous iron: a randomized controlled study. J Am Coll Cardiol 2001;37:1775–80.
37. Mancini DM, Katz SD, Lang CC, et al. Effect of erythropoietin on exercise capacity in patients with moderate to severe chronic heart failure. Circulation 2003;107:294–9.
38. Abraham W, Klapholz M, Anand I, et al. The effect of darbepoetin alfa treatment on clinical outcomes in anemic patients with symptomatic heart failure: a proplanned pooled analysis of two randomized, double-blind placebo-controlled trials. Eur J Heart Fail 2006;27:166–7.
39. Ponikowski P, Anker SD, Szachniewicz, et al. Effect of darbepoetin alfa on exercise tolerance in anemic patients with symptomatic chronic heart failure: a randomized, double-blind, placebo-controlled trial. J Am Coll Cardiol 2007;49:753–62.
40. van Veldhuisen DJ, Dickstein K, Cohen-Solal A, et al. Randomized, double-blind, placebo-controlled study to evaluate the effect of two dosing regimens of darepoetin alfa in patients with heart failure and anaemia. Eur Heart J 2007;28:2208–16.
41. Ghali JK, Anand IS, Abraham WT, et al. On behalf of the study of anemia in heart failure trial (Stamina-HeFT) group. Randomized double-blind trial of darbepoetin alfa in patients with symptomatic heart failure and anemia. Circulation 2008;117:526–35.
42. Parissis JT, Kourea K, Panou F, et al. Effects of darbepoetin alpha on right and left ventricular systolic and diastolic function in anemic patients with chronic heart failure secondary to ischemic or idiopathic dilated cardiomyopathy. Am Heart J 2008;155(4):751, e1–7.
43. van Veldhuisen DJ, Dickstein K, Cohen-Solal A, et al. Randomized, double-blind, placebo-controlled study to evaluate the effect of two dosing regimens of darbepoetin alfa in patients with heart failure and anaemia. Eur Heart J 2007;28(18):2208–16.

44. Palazzuoli A, Silverberg D, Iovine F, et al. Erythro-poietin improves anemia exercise tolerance and renal function and reduces B-type natriuretic peptide and hospitalization in patients with heart failure and anemia. Am Heart J 2006;152(6): 1096.e9–15.

45. Tang WHW, Tong W, Jain A, et al. Evaluation and long-term prognosis of new-onset transient, and persistent anemia in ambulatory patients with chronic heart failure. J Am Coll Cardiol 2008;51: 569–76.

46. van der Meer P, Groenveld HF, Januzzi JL, et al. Erythropoietin treatment in patients with chronic heart failure: a meta-analysis. Heart 2009;95: 1309–14.

47. Geisler BP, van Dam RM, Gazelle GS, et al. Risk of bias in meta-analysis on erythropoietin-stimulating agents in heart failure. Heart 2009;95:1278–9.

48. Parfrey PS, Foley RN, Wittreich BH, et al. Double-blind comparison of full and partial anemia correction in inci-dent hemodialysis patients without symptomatic heart disease. J Am Soc Nephrol 2005;16:2180–9.

49. Zhang Y, Thamer M, Stefanik K, et al. Epoetin requirements predict mortality in hemodialysis patients. Am J Kidney Dis 2004;44:866–76.

50. Servilla KS, Singh AK, Hunt WC, et al. Anemia management and association of race with mortality and hospitalization in a large not-for-profit dialysis organization. Am J Kidney Dis 2009;54:498–510.

51. Wang O, Kilpatrick RD, Critchlow CW, et al. Relation-ship between epoetin alfa dose and mortality: find-ings from a marginal structural model. Clin J Am Soc Nephrol 2010;5:182–8.

52. Streja E, Kovesdy CP, Greenland S, et al. Erythropoi-etin, iron depletion, and relative thrombocytosis: a possible explanation for hemoglobin-survival paradox in hemodialysis. Am J Kidney Dis 2008; 52:727–36.

53. Bradbury BD, Wang O, Critchlow CW, et al. Exploring relative mortality and epoetin alfa dose among hemodialysis patients. Am J Kidney Dis 2008;51:62–70.

54. Zhang Y, Thamer M, Cotter D, et al. Estimated effect of epoetin dosage on survival among elderly hemo-dialysis patients in the United States. Clin J Am Soc Nephrol 2009;4:638–44.

55. Szczech LA, Barnhart HX, Sapp S, et al. A secondary analysis of the CHOIR trial shows that comorbid conditions differentially affect outcomes during anemia treatment. Kidney Int 2010;77:239–46.

Epidemiology of Cardiorenal Syndrome

Robert J. Mentz, MD[a], Eldrin F. Lewis, MD, MPH[b],*

KEYWORDS

- Cardiorenal syndrome • Congestive heart failure
- Epidemiology • Management • End-of-life

The prevalence of symptomatic chronic heart failure (CHF) in the United States is estimated at 2% in those over 45 years of age with a lifetime risk of CHF estimated at 20%.[1,2] CHF is the leading cause of hospitalization in persons over age 65. Responsible for more than 1 million hospitalizations annually in the United States, CHF costs were approximately $37 billion in 2009.[3,4] In trying to improve the management of these complicated patients, the interactions between the heart and the kidney have become an area of considerable interest.[5] The presence of renal impairment is common in low and preserved ejection fraction (EF) as well as symptomatic and asymptomatic patients.[6,7] Renal dysfunction plays an important role in the progression of cardiovascular disease[8–10] and serves as an independent risk factor for morbidity and mortality in patients with heart failure (HF).[11,12] In end-stage renal disease patients, approximately 30% have CHF on initiation of dialysis[13] and patients commonly die from cardiovascular causes.[14] This interdependence of the heart and the kidney has been captured in Ronco and colleagues'[15] recent definition of the cardiorenal syndrome (CRS) **(Table 1)**. The CRS includes acute and chronic conditions where the heart or the kidney serves as the primary failing organ with resulting dysfunction in both organs perpetuating the combined dysfunction through interrelated neurohormonal and hemodynamic mechanisms.[15] This definition encompasses multiple entities that have previously been reviewed in the literature separately (HF or

renal failure, worsening renal function [WRF], and diuretic resistance) and provides structure for addressing acute and longitudinal care.

This review discusses potential pathophysiologic mechanisms of the CRS; its epidemiology; inpatient and long-term care, including investigational therapies and mechanical fluid removal; and end-of-life and palliative care.

PATHOPHYSIOLOGY AND RISK FACTORS FOR CRS

Several recent reviews summarize current understanding of the pathophysiology of CRS.[14,16,17] These articles focus largely on renal insufficiency secondary to HF (CRS types I and II). Briefly, a decrease in systolic or diastolic cardiac function results in hemodynamic derangements, including low cardiac output and arterial underfilling, which are initially compensated by mechanisms of sodium retention and vasoconstriction (eg, renin-angiotensin-aldosterone system [RAAS], sympathetic nervous system, tubuloglomerular feedback [TGF], endothelin, and vasopressin) balanced with activation of vasodilatory (eg, nitric oxide, bradykinin, and prostaglandins), natriuretic, and cytokine systems.[14,16–18] These compensatory mechanisms become imbalanced due to blunting of reflexes (eg, atrial-renal) and unchecked control mechanisms (eg, lack of "escape" from salt-retaining effects of aldosterone nonosmotic release of arginine vasopressin [AVP], and elevated adenosine-mediated afferent arteriole vasoconstriction

a Department of Internal Medicine, Brigham and Women's Hospital, 75 Francis Street, Boston, MA 02115, USA
b Cardiovascular Division, Department of Medicine, Brigham and Women's Hospital, 75 Francis Street, Boston, MA 02115, USA
* Corresponding author.
E-mail address: eflewis@partners.org

Heart Failure Clin 6 (2010) 333–346
doi:10.1016/j.hfc.2010.03.001
1551-7136/10/$ – see front matter © 2010 Elsevier Inc. All rights reserved.

Table 1
Cardiorenal syndrome

Type I: acute CRS

Abrupt worsening of cardiac function
  (eg, acute cardiogenic shock or ADHF)
  leading to acute kidney injury

Type II: chronic CRS

Chronic abnormalities in cardiac function
  (eg, CHF) causing progressive and potentially
  permanent CKD

Type III: acute renocardiac syndrome

Abrupt worsening of renal function
  (eg, acute kidney ischemia or
  glomerulonephritis) causing acute cardiac
  disorder (eg, HF, arrhythmia, ischemia)

Type IV: chronic renocardiac syndrome

CKD (eg, chronic glomerular or interstitial
  disease) contributing to decreased cardiac
  function, cardiac hypertrophy, or increased
  risk of adverse cardiovascular events

Type V: secondary CRS

Systemic condition (eg, DM, sepsis) causing
  cardiac and renal dysfunction

Data from Jessup M, Costanzo MR. The cardiorenal syndrome: do we need a change of strategy or a change of tactics? J Am Coll Cardiol 2009;53(7):597–9; and Ronco C, Haapio M, House AA, et al. Cardiorenal syndrome. J Am Coll Cardiol 2008;52(19):1527–39.

via TGF) in the setting of structural changes (eg, aldosterone-induced myocardial fibrosis and renovascular changes).[18,19] As a result, these maladaptive mechanisms promote a vicious cycle increasing preload and afterload and also causing oxidative stress, inflammation, and chronic renal hypoxia with resultant adverse effects on cardiac and renal function.[14,15,20] Elevated levels of cytokines, including tumor necrosis factor (TNF)-α, interleukin (IL)-1, and IL-6, in HF patients are associated with the progression of CRS via effects on negative inotropy, cardiac remodeling, and ischemic acute kidney injury.[14,15] Concomitant liver dysfunction may also play a prominent role because dysregulation of the hepatorenal reflex, vasoactive mediator-induced circulatory dysfunction, and decreased hepatic clearance of cytokines exacerbate renal and cardiac function.[21]

CRS cannot be explained by the traditional argument of poor forward flow or prerenal physiology with overdiuresis. WRF does not seem to be associated with reduced EF or poor forward flow as observed in retrospective studies[22,23] and database analysis,[24] or directly from hemodynamic data.[25] As demonstrated in the Evaluation Study of Congestive Heart Failure and Pulmonary Artery Catheterization Effectiveness (ESCAPE) evaluating hemodynamics via pulmonary artery (PA) catheters in patients with acute decompensated HF (ADHF), cardiac output was not associated with baseline renal dysfunction or the development of WRF.[25] The only hemodynamic parameter associated with renal function was right atrial pressure. Renal dysfunction is more likely to result from raised renal vein pressure than hypoperfusion.[18] Renal perfusion depends on the difference between arterial and venous pressures, known as transrenal perfusion pressure. A growing body of literature supports the prominent role of venous congestion in WRF. Mullens and colleagues[26] used PA catheter data from 145 patients with ADHF to demonstrate that venous congestion is the most important hemodynamic factor driving WRF. Impaired cardiac output on admission and improvement in cardiac output after therapy had little impact on WRF in typical (ie, noncardiogenic shock) patients with ADHF. In contrast, higher admission central venous pressure (CVP) predicted WRF independent of baseline renal dysfunction and was associated with severity of WRF.[26] Elevated CVP has been shown to have adverse effects on sodium excretion (via stimulation of the RAAS) and renal hemodynamics with reduction in estimated glomerular filtration rate (eGFR) and renal blood flow, perhaps resulting in renal hypoxia.[16,17,26] The reduction in venous renal congestion by diuretics is a proposed mechanism for improvement in creatinine during ADHF management.

Recent data question the validity of concerns about diuretic use resulting in intravascular volume depletion (ie, prerenal physiology) during early ADHF management.[27] Patients admitted with ADHF commonly experience WRF early in their course when they are still volume overloaded rather than after aggressive diuresis.[27] When markedly volume overloaded, these patients are able to protect their intravascular volume by rapid redistribution from the extravascular compartment.[17] Although overdiuresis can eventually result in intravascular volume depletion with an elevation in creatinine and serum urea nitrogen (SUN), prerenal physiology likely does not play a major role in the early development of CRS.

Baseline renal insufficiency seems a strong independent risk factor for the development of WRF in systolic and diastolic HF.[6,22,23,28–31] Other risk factors include a history of hypertension (HTN)[25,28–31] and diabetes mellitus (DM).[6,25,28,30,32] Additional risk factors for WRF that have been reported in several retrospective analyses include older age,[22,32] a history of HF,[30,31] coronary artery disease or an ischemic etiology of CHF,[22,28] and pulmonary edema on chest radiograph or examination.[23,29] These risk factors along with others need to be validated in prospective randomized controlled trials. Although ESCAPE supported the risk factors of DM and HTN in the development of WRF, it did not independently link baseline renal function with an increased risk of development of WRF.[25] Nonetheless, even though there have been significant increases in HTN and DM with time, the incidence of WRF has not been observed to increase,[28] possibly due to changes in clinical practice and more judicious monitoring of renal function during treatment for ADHF. Thus, the conceptual model that simply having long-standing HTN, DM, and CHF results in poor forward flow and chronic kidney disease (CKD) and predisposes HF patients to WRF has not been proved. More likely, underlying DM, HTN, CHF, CKD, and other factors create a maladapative neurohormonal milieu on top of chronic systemic structural changes that culminate with increased risk for WRF that depends on the variable contribution of each of these factors in individual patients.

In addition to the baseline patient characteristics, treatment factors linked to WRF have been evaluated in several studies. Butler and colleagues[30] showed that angiotensin-converting enzyme (ACE) doses during hospitalization for ADHF are not independently associated with WRF. Jose and colleagues[33] used data from the Survival and Ventricular Enlargement (SAVE) trial involving 2231 patients with systolic dysfunction after myocardial infarction to show that ACE inhibitor use was not associated with the development of WRF. Thus, some clinicians tolerate a slight increase in creatinine to initiate proved RAAS inhibition due to documented morbidity and mortality benefits. Butler and colleagues[30] demonstrated that patients who developed WRF received higher doses of loop diuretics on the day before WRF. Similarly, Cowie and colleagues[23] found that patients who experienced WRF did not have larger outpatient loop diuretic doses, but they received higher max doses while in the hospital. ESCAPE demonstrated that in-hospital thiazide use but not loop diuretic dose was a risk factor for WRF.[25] Because diuretics activate the RAAS system and worsen the neurohormonal environment, it is appealing to incriminate their use in WRF. It is currently not known, however, whether or not diuretics have a causal relationship with WRF or if higher doses are a marker of more severe underlying disease characterized by greater diuretic resistance. Diuretic-free regimens with use of

ultrafiltration (UF) are being studied for acute decompensated CHF patients.

The clinical observation of decreased diuretic responsiveness or diuretic resistance reveals additional potential mechanisms of CRS. In HF patients, gut hypoperfusion and edema may necessitate intravenous diuretic administration due to decreased absorption. Furthermore, protein binding of loop diuretics results in an increased volume of distribution in hypoalbuminemic CHF patients and the organic acids present in renal failure inhibit the tubular secretion of diuretics.[17] Moreover, diuretic braking (with post-diuretic sodium retention) and chronic diuretic therapy-induced tubular cell hypertrophy result in enhanced sodium reuptake culminating in decreased responsiveness.[15,17]

In developing an approach to predict which patients are more likely to experience CRS, the authors remain confined to the largely unrevealing list of common comorbidities in HF patients: older, hypertensive diabetics with a history of HF and baseline renal insufficiency who receive more loop diuretics. More work is required to identify these patients earlier during management, which may enable more aggressive volume reduction and decreased length of stay.

THE EPIDEMIOLOGY OF CHRONIC CRS

Moderate to severe CKD (defined as eGFR <60 mL/min/1.73 m^2; stage III CKD) is present in 20% to 60% of HF outpatients and is associated with substantial morbidity and mortality (using the World Health Organization's anemia criteria of a hemoglobin level [below 13 g/dL in men and below 12 g/dL in women]). These estimates primarily are limited to type II and type IV CRS involving chronic abnormalities in cardiac or renal function causing progressive CKD and decreased cardiac function, respectively. These prevalence values are likely underestimated, especially type IV CRS, given the under-representation of elderly patients and those with moderate to severe renal dysfunction in the heterogenous HF studies. The Studies of Left Ventricular Dysfunction (SOLVD) revealed baseline prevalence of at least moderate CKD in 20.6% of patients in the prevention trial and 35.7% in the treatment trial but excluded patients with serum creatinine greater than 2 mg/dL or age over 79.[7] Moderate CKD was associated with an increase in all-cause mortality largely explained by an increased risk for pump failure.[7] Excluding patients with a serum creatinine greater than 3 mg/dL, the Candesartan in Heart Failure—Assessment of Reduction in Mortality and Morbidity (CHARM) and Digoxin

Intervention Group (DIG) studies reported prevalence values of 36% and 46% for moderate CKD, respectively.[6,12] The DIG trial reported a threshold mortality effect with a steep increase in annual mortality when eGFR decreased below 50 mL/min/1.73 m^2.[12] In contrast, the CHARM study demonstrated a stepwise increase in mortality and admission risk with reducing eGFR.[6] Furthermore, CHARM revealed that eGFR is an independent predictor of mortality in patients with preserved EF.[6] Substudies from the Second Prospective Randomized Study of Ibopamine on Mortality and Efficacy (PRIME-II) indicated that eGFR was the strongest predictor of mortality (ie, stronger than EF).[11,34] The lowest quintile of eGFR in their study (<44 mL/min/1.73 m^2) had a nearly 3-fold risk of mortality.[11] The prevalence values for moderate CKD women and elderly blacks are 54% and 57%, respectively.[35,36] Data from specialized ambulatory CHF clinics report a prevalence of approximately 60%.[37,38] The population-based studies are thus a better indicator of the true prevalence of moderate CKD in the outpatient CHF population (reflecting a percentage of type II and IV CRS), which is likely at least 40% to 50%. Data from the Framingham Heart Study and the Rochester Epidemiology Project in Olmsted County indicate that for incident HF cases, the average eGFR was 58.2 mL/min and the average creatinine was 1.6 mg/dL, respectively,[39,40] suggestive of moderate renal insufficiency on average in the HF community.

In their meta-analysis of HF studies with greater than or equal to 1-year follow-up, Smith and colleagues[41] report that the mortality rate was 51% in those with moderate to severe renal impairment versus 24% in those with normal renal function. Mortality increased incrementally across the range of renal function, suggesting a dose-response relationship.[41] Specifically, there was a 15% increased mortality risk for every 0.5 mg/dL increase in creatinine or a 7% increased risk for every 10 mL/min decrease in eGFR.[41] Similarly, data from the Acute Decompensated Heart Failure National Registry (ADHERE) revealed increased in-hospital mortality and length of stay with increasing stage of CKD.[24] Normal renal function was associated with an in-hospital mortality of 1.9% and length of stay of 5.3 days versus 7.6% and 7 days in stage IV kidney disease. Also, more severe kidney dysfunction was associated with increased mechanical ventilation, more frequent ICU admission and a greater incidence of cardiopulmonary resuscitation.[24] Thus, baseline renal insufficiency represents one of the strongest predictors of morbidity and mortality in HF patients with low and preserved EF.

THE EPIDEMIOLOGY OF ACUTE CRS

In trying to capture the prevalence of CRS in hospitalized patients, previous reports focused on renal dysfunction on admission for HF and WRF, which largely reflect type I and III CRS. This eliminated inpatient changes that may influence renal function, such as contrast exposure, overdiuresis, or dynamic changes in renal perfusion due to vasoactive medicines or transient low-flow states. The ADHERE registry revealed that 63.6% of ADHF patients had at least moderate renal insufficiency on admission.[24] The mean admission creatinine has increased over time from 1.46 mg/dL in 1987 to 1.62 mg/dL in 2002.[28] This increase in creatinine corresponds to a decrease in eGFR (from 73 mL/min/1.73 m^2 to 55 mL/min/1.73 m^2) consistent with stage III CKD. With the use of advanced medical therapy and defibrillators decreasing sudden cardiac death, future admissions may involve a significantly larger population of elderly adults and those with advanced CHF and likely higher admission creatinine.

During inpatient hospitalization, WRF occurs frequently and is a subset of acute CRS. Initial studies of acute CRS used various definitions of WRF.[22,23,25,29–31] A widely accepted definition is creatinine elevation greater than or equal to 0.3 mg/dL, a threshold that has maximum sensitivity and specificity for in-hospital mortality and length of stay.[27] WRF develops early in the course of ADHF hospitalization, often within the first 3 days,[30,31] with an incidence range from 20% to 30%.[22,23,29,31] These reports are now supported by the first prospective trial in ESCAPE where the incidence was 29.5%.[25] Studies show that WRF is associated with an increased length of stay of 2 days on average,[29,30] a 2-fold higher in-hospital complication rate,[31] increased hospital costs,[29] a 3-fold increase in mortality during hospitalization,[29] an increased 6-month mortality rate (43% versus 36% in those without WRF; odds ratio for mortality of 1.62 with 95% CI of 1.45–1.82)[42] and increased mortality out to 5 years.[28] By showing that an increase in creatinine of as little as 0.2 mg/dL is associated with increased 6-month mortality, Smith and colleagues[43] revealed the prognostic importance of even small increases in creatinine. WRF seems to have associations with outcome, including in patients admitted with normal creatinine, regardless of peak creatinine and discharge values.[31,43]

In addition to baseline renal insufficiency and WRF, SUN has been recently demonstrated to have prognostic significance. Fonarow and colleagues[44] used data from the ADHERE registry to show that admission SUN greater than 43 mg/dL is the best predictor of in-hospital mortality in patients with ADHF. SUN had greater predictive power than elevated serum creatinine. Klein and colleagues[45] extended the usefulness of SUN by revealing that the change in SUN during hospitalization had the most important impact on 60-day mortality. Hemodynamic changes involving activation of the RAAS and AVP-induced SUN reabsorption in the collecting duct have been postulated as mechanisms to explain the usefulness of SUN.[16]

EXPLANATIONS FOR INCREASED MORTALITY

In addition to the pathophysiologic derangement (discussed previously), many different explanations for the increase in morbidity and mortality with renal dysfunction in HF are posited in the literature. First, renal dysfunction has been shown to limit the use of medications, such as ACE inhibitors, angiotensin receptor blocker (ARBs), and β-blockers, due to concerns about exacerbating renal function or causing hyperkalemia, especially in the elderly.[19,40–48] Also, patients with renal dysfunction have greater comorbid illnesses, such as peripheral vascular disease, dyslipidemia, and anemia.[49] The anemia of CKD is associated with poor outcome.[50,51] Al Ahmad and colleagues[50] used data from the Studies of Left Ventricular Dysfunction (SOLVD) database to show that for every decrease in hematocrit of 1%, the mortality rate increased by 2.7%. Data from large prospective trials of CKD patients (with and without HF), however, have failed to show a benefit from treating such anemia.[52,53] Renal dysfunction also leads to abnormal calcium and phosphate metabolism with secondary hyperparathyroidism, which may have a role in abnormal vascular calcifications and arterial stiffness.[54–59] Additional explanations include elevated procoagulant biomarkers (eg, hyperhomocysteinemia),[60,61] albuminuria,[62] and uremic toxins (eg, indoxyl sulfate[63]) as well as hyponatremia[64] and other electrolyte disturbances with resultant increased arrhythmia risk.[65]

ACUTE MANAGEMENT

The first steps in the management of CRS include prevention and anticipation. Avoidance of nephrotoxic agents, including iodinated contrasts, certain higher risk antibiotics, and nonsteroidal anti-inflammatory drugs, should be undertaken whenever possible.[17] Anticipation of CRS involves early estimation of GFR via the modification of diet in renal disease equation as well as consideration of other suspected risk factors (discussed previously). Nonetheless, early diagnosis of CRS is a challenge with classic markers, such as creatinine and eGFR, which may take days to become elevated. Novel biomarkers, including serum neutrophil gelatinase-associated lipocalin (NGAL), urine IL-18, and kidney injury molecule-1 (KIM-1) may allow for earlier detection of kidney injury in the future[18] because elevation may occur much earlier in the time course of kidney injury (<12 hours) in comparison with creatinine.[15]

Once diagnosis of CRS is established, early management should involve symptom control and optimization of standard HF therapy.[17] Early symptom relief includes medications, such as diuretics and morphine for congestive symptoms, and may involve procedures, such as paracentesis and thoracentesis. Patients should be sodium and fluid restricted (<1000 mL per 24 hours of free water especially if hyponatremic[20]). Accurate daily weight is critical, because body weight is an indicator while managing CRS.[20] Early optimization of blood pressure and vasodilator therapy as well as adjuvant therapies, such as digoxin and cardiac resynchronization therapy (CRT), remains key.[17]

Despite limited trial data, diuretics have long been an essential part of CHF management. Diuretic therapy may have harmful effects on the progression of CRS, including exacerbating neurohormonal activity, worsening left ventricular (LV) function, and inducing hypovolemia and electrolyte abnormalities.[16,20] Until prospective, randomized trials with adequate power are performed to evaluate their optimization in the management of CRS, reliance is on knowledge about the principles of loop diuretics. First, consider drug half-life and the lack of a smooth dose-response curve such that a threshold level is required for diuretic effect.[17] Consequently, the dose may need to be doubled until the appropriate response occurs. Although most studies to date evaluating bolus versus continuous infusion have been small crossover trials with heterogenous populations, a Cochrane review suggests that continuous infusion of loop diuretics may provide greater diuresis, a better safety profile (less tinnitus or hearing loss), and possibly shorter length of stay and lower cardiac mortality.[66] During diuresis, patients should be closely monitored for hypotension, electrolyte depletion, and arrhythmias. Combination therapy with thiazides has been shown to increase diuretic responsiveness but careful monitoring is required due to an increased risk of hyponatremia, hypokalemia, metabolic alkalosis, and dehydration.[18] There have been reports of improved diuretic responsiveness with rotation between different loop diuretics[16] and the use of salt-poor albumin infusion in an attempt to deliver more diuretic to the kidney,[20] but future randomized trial data are needed to validate these approaches.

Although ACE inhibitors and ARBs result in significant mortality reduction in CHF, their association with worsening GFR makes continuation of their use in CRS a common clinical dilemma.[18] Trials of these neurohormonal antagonists typically excluded those with baseline renal dysfunction. Of the available trial data, there have been few subgroup analyses of those with renal dysfunction. The Cooperative North Scandinavian Enalapril Survival Study (CONSENSUS) evaluating the longitudinal use of enalapril in New York Heart Association (NYHA) class IV CHF revealed a similar risk reduction in those with renal impairment compared with those without.[18] Of the scarce data available on the use of ACE inhibitors in CHF patients who experience WRF, an association between ACE inhibitor use and WRF has not been demonstrated.[30,33] Therefore, a reasonable approach is to continue ACE inhibition despite a rise in creatinine unless renal function steadily declines or hyperkalemia develops.[67]

The onset of action for spironolactone is slower than with loop diuretics and the peak effect occurs at 48 hours.[16] The risk of hyperkalemia is of great concern with their use in the setting of CRS. Recommendations are to use mineralocorticoid antagonists with caution in those with reduced eGFR and to avoid this class when eGFR falls below 30 mL/min/1.73 m². [67] The 2 large trials that demonstrated the reduction in mortality in CHF with mineralocorticoid antagonists also did not use natriuretic doses.[67] Future trials are required to evaluate the use of mineralocorticoid antagonists in the acute setting.

Although there is limited literature specifically evaluating the use of β-blockers in those with CRS, post hoc analyses of randomized data from Outcomes of a Prospective Trial of Intravenous Milrinone for Exacerbations of Chronic Heart Failure (OPTIME-CHF), the Carvedilol or Metoprolol European Trial (COMET), and ESCAPE as well as registry data from the Organized Program to Initiate Lifesaving Treatment in Hospitalized Patients with Heart Failure (OPTIMIZE-HF) demonstrate that β-blocker withdrawal during admission for ADHF is associated with increased mortality.[68–71] The initiation or continuation of β-blocker therapy resulted in reduced mortality and readmission when compared with no β-blocker use in eligible patients.[71] Furthermore, β-blocker withdrawal was independently associated with a greater than 2-fold increased risk of death.[71] Continuation of β-blocker therapy was well

tolerated after discharge and substantially more patients were treated as outpatients as a consequence of in-hospital continuation.[71] Medication prescription at the time of discharge has been shown the strongest predictor of long-term use.[72] Recommendations are to continue beta blockade unless patients experience hemodynamic instability. Further randomized, prospective studies are needed to determine whether or not withdrawal of β-blockers is associated with increased risk beyond that of not receiving benefit from longitudinal use.

Renal-dose dopamine should not be used routinely in CRS management. Although several early studies showed improved kidney function with increased diuresis and natriuresis,[17] the consensus among studies with rigorous methodology is that low-dose dopamine for the treatment or prevention of ARF cannot be justified.[17] Inotropic support should be guided by the underlying physiology with or without hemodynamic guidance. Nesiritide is a recombinant analog of human brain natriuretic peptide, which seems to produce vasodilation as its main effect.[17] Early nesiritide trials and a large prospective registry suggested that nesiritide was safe in short-term management of ADHF, albeit with conflicting results on its effects on renal function, natriuresis, and diuresis.[17] In 2005, a meta-analysis of randomized, double-blind, placebo-controlled trials suggested that nesiritide may have an adverse impact on renal function (presumably by way of systemic hypotension) and may increase mortality.[73] In contrast, a meta-analysis by Arora and colleagues[74] showed no increased mortality with nesiritide.[74] The studies that demonstrated negative outcomes used nesiritide at higher doses than those currently recommended. Subsequent studies have suggested that nesiritide may have renal-protective effects when used at appropriate doses in inpatient and outpatient settings.[17] The ongoing Acute Study of Clinical Effectiveness of Nesiritide in Subjects With Decompensated Heart Failure (ASCEND-HF) may answer some of the questions on the appropriate use of nesiritide in hospitalized patients with ADHF.[75] Systematic review of the use of inotropes in acute and CHF suggests a negative impact on survival except in a few patients with severe "low output failure."[20] Therefore, because inotropic therapy may have harmful effects on the progression of CRS by further augmenting neurohormonal activation,[17] future studies need to clarify any potential use outside of maintenance of blood pressure in hemodynamically unstable patients.

The investigational therapies of vasopressin and adenosine antagonists have been shown to have positive effects on fluid loss as well as symptoms and may possibly reduce key endpoints in the case of adenosine antagonists. Vasopressin antagonists block renal water resorption (via the V2 receptor in the distal tubule and collecting duct) and vasoconstriction (V1a subtype in vascular smooth muscle cells), resulting in aquaresis, increased sodium concentration, reduced peripheral resistance and mean arterial pressure, and inhibition of AVP-mediated cardiomyocyte hypertrophy.[17] The Study of Ascending Levels of Tolvaptan in Hyponatremia (SALT) 1 and 2 showed that use of 1 of these agents (tolvaptan, a V2 antagonist) can raise serum sodium levels in patients with CHF.[76] The Efficacy of Vasopressin Antagonism in Heart Failure Outcome Study with Tolvaptan (EVEREST), which studied tolvaptan in combination with standard therapy (including diuretics) demonstrated modest effects on weight and symptoms (dyspnea and edema) in the acute setting but there was no long-term benefit on major clinical outcomes, including mortality or hospitalization.[77,78] There were no differences in renal function with the addition of tolvaptan to optimal medical therapy. Although hyponatremia in HF has been shown to correlate with mortality,[64] the use of aquaretics, such as vasopressin antagonist, have thus far have not been shown to reduce mortality and are, therefore, unlikely to play a major role in future management of acute CRS.

A1 adenosine antagonists have the potential to disrupt the TGF loop (which results in afferent arteriole vasoconstriction and decreased GFR) with potential positive effects on renal function and diuretic resistance.[17] Also, they may have beneficial inotropic effects by blocking adenosine's negative inotropic effects on cardiac A1 receptors.[17] Several small studies have shown that A1 antagonists may preserve renal function during diuresis while promoting enhanced response to loop diuretics.[17] Pilot results of the Placebo-controlled Randomized Study of the Selective A_1 Adenosine Receptor Antagonist Rolofylline for Patients Hospitalized with Acute Heart Failure and Volume Overload to Assess Treatment Effect on Congestion and Renal Function (PROTECT) support the use of 1 of these agents in patients with ADHF and renal impairment or diuretic resistance.[79] Rolofylline resulted in more rapid weight loss and a suggestion of reduced dyspnea, WRF, and 60-day mortality or readmission for cardiovascular or renal causes.[79] The larger follow-up study, however, did not show efficacy with this agent and future research is required.

UF offers another approach to fluid removal in the setting of volume overload, diuretic resistance, and WRF. UF harnesses a transmembrane pressure gradient to filter plasma water across a semipermeable membrane.[17] The rationale for the use of UF is based on its rapidity of fluid removal, degree of sodium clearance, and avoidance of maladaptive autoregulatory responses.[80] UF has been shown to remove more sodium and less potassium than diuretics for an equivalent volume.[17] If the removal rate and plasma-refill rate are appropriately balanced, then activation of RAAS and hypotension can be avoided.[81,82] UF may also be able to clear large biologic molecules (eg, cytokines, such as TNF-α and interleukins) that have an adverse role in the pathophysiology of HF.[80] Whether or not UF prevents WRF or improves hard endpoints in patients with CRS is unclear. Initial studies were of small sample size, included highly selected patient populations, did not report the incidence of WRF, and had short follow-up and it was unclear whether or not the patients were resistant to aggressive diuretic regimens.[17] One study showed that despite large fluid removal via UF, 50% of the patients ultimately required hemodialysis (HD) and the length of stay, costs, and mortality rates were high.[83] The Ultrafiltration versus IV Diuretics for Patients Hospitalized for Acute Decompensated Congestive Heart Failure (UNLOAD) study, a larger randomized trial of UF (n = 200), demonstrated greater fluid loss and reduced length of stay and readmission with UF compared with diuresis, but no protective effect of UF on renal function was observed.[84] Moreover, the study patient population seemed more stable than typical patients with ADHF and the groups were not controlled for the total amount of volume loss.[80] Further randomized trial data are required to support the use of UF.

The use of peritoneal dialysis (PD) in the management of treatment-resistant CHF has not been studied extensively, yet small studies report significant benefits. PD has been shown to restore diuretic responsiveness, decrease pulmonary HTN, improve NYHA class and quality of life, reduce length of stay, and substantially reduce hospitalizations.[82] As presented by Krishnan and Oreopoulos,[85] PD is associated with preservation of renal function, gentle continuous ultrafiltration, hemodynamic stability, maintenance of normonatremia, better middle-molecule clearance, and perhaps less inflammation than HD. The theory of peritoneal clearance of middle molecules or myocardium-depressing substances, such as TNF-α, ANP, myocardial depressing factor, and IL-1 and IL-6,[86] is appealing but requires further investigation. Kazory and Ross[80] elegantly discuss how the mass clearance of these compounds is low, they have short half-life periods, and they can rapidly reappear. Furthermore, the nonspecific nature of clearance means that beneficial cytokines are also lost.[80] PD offers volume removal without the rapid fall in blood pressure possible with UF.[82] In comparison with HD, PD does not require vascular access or heparin. Moreover, PD is already established as a long-term, home-based therapy and does not required complex machinery or hospital resources. Recently, use of icodextrin-containing solutions has allowed for sustained PD over longer dwell periods. The longer dwells may allow for maintenance of euvolemia in CHF patients with 1 overnight exchange.[82] Extended dwells also likely reduce peritoneal infection risks given the small number of bag changes.[82]

Registry data in ESRD patients with CHF on PD demonstrated increased mortality with PD versus HD, thereby increasing controversy over its use.[87] The data from this registry were from 1995 to 1997, when automated PD and icodextrin solutions were less available.[82] Couchoud and colleagues[88] demonstrated similar survival rates for PD and HD in a group of 3512 patients, but there was still an increased risk of mortality with PD versus HD. Increased mortality risk in patients treated with PD may be counterbalanced by overall satisfaction, independence, and better quality of life.[89,90] Randomized trials of PD are required to further investigate its role in CRS management.

LONGITUDINAL CARE

Appropriate prescription of medications known to reduce mortality in CHF remains central to longitudinal care. Physician concerns of WRF and hyperkalemia result in underuse of medications known to reduce mortality, such as ACE inhibitors, ARBs, and spironolactone.[19,46–48] In the general HF population, prehospital cardiac regimens contained an ACE inhibitor or ARB only 53% of the time, and 48% of patients were on a β-blocker.[91] After hospitalization, only 69% were prescribed an ACE inhibitor or ARB and 59% received β-blockers.[91] In ESRD patients with LV dysfunction, 72% received β-blockade, 36% ACE inhibition, and only 25.5% the combination.[92] When appropriately titrated and monitored, these medications can be safely administered to CKD patients with similar benefits to the general population.[93] One meta-analysis demonstrated that up to a 30% increase in creatinine with ACE inhibitors that stabilizes within 2 months is associated with long-term nephroprotection.[94] Data from the CONSENSUS trial support that those patients who experience a rise in creatinine after ACE initiation may be the subgroup who achieve the greatest benefit from their use.[95] Although one-third of patients with severe HF experience a substantial increase (>30%) in creatinine with initiation of ACE inhibitors, only a small fraction of patients requires discontinuation of therapy, and creatinine levels return to baseline in most patients even without dose adjustment.[96] Severely increased creatinine that does not stabilize could point to the possibility of underlying renovascular disease, particularly in the elderly.[97] In patients with moderate or severe renal insufficiency, therapy with ACE inhibitors should be initiated at a low dose and gradually up-titrated with careful monitoring of renal function and electrolytes.[67] Dynamic changes in renal function require intensification of monitoring.

None of the large clinical trials of β-blockers in HF has reported subgroup analyses based on renal function. One observational study evaluating β-blockers in post–myocardial infarction patients with ventricular dysfunction demonstrated a similar survival benefit in patients with creatinine greater than or less than 2 mg/dL.[98] Several studies have shown that the initiation of β-blockers may lead to initial worsening of renal function but that as cardiac function improves, renal function also improves.[18] Long-term treatment with β-blockers results in significant improvements in renal function and anemia.[18] Implications for the use of β-blockers in patients with renal dysfunction include special consideration for those that are renally excreted (atenolol, nadalol, and sotalol) versus hepatically cleared (metoprolol and carvedilol).

Data on the use of aldosterone antagonists in renal insufficiency are limited. The Randomized Aldactone Evaluation Study (RALES) demonstrated a 30% mortality reduction in patients with severe HF but excluded patients with a creatinine greater than 2.5 mg/dL.[99] The risk of hyperkalemia with aldosterone antagonists requires that renal function and electrolytes be carefully monitored. Suggestions are to avoid spironolactone in patients with a GFR less than 30 mL/min/1.73 m^2 and to use them cautiously in patients with a GFR of 30 to 60 mL/min/1.73 m^2 and at doses no higher than 25 mg daily.[67]

Digitalis does not affect CHF survival but it has been shown to result in a 28% reduction in HF hospitalizations.[100] The clearance of digitalis varies linearly with GFR such that renal dysfunction may affect its safety.[67] When used in patients with renal dysfunction, the loading dose and frequency of dosing must be modified.[67] No studies have evaluated whether or not the effects of digitalis on clinical outcomes differ by renal function.

Cardiac transplantation and left ventricular assist device (LVAD) therapy have traditionally had low clinical applicability for the majority of

CRS patients given their advanced age, high surgical risk, poor prognosis, and comorbidities that preclude them from consideration.[20,101] End-organ dysfunction, such as renal insufficiency, is associated with poor outcome after LVAD implantation.[102] GFR, however, has not consistently been shown an independent predictor of outcome in multivariate models, suggesting that use of GFR alone as a contraindication to invasive therapy is not data driven.[102] LVAD therapy has demonstrated improvements in renal function even in the absence of pre-existing low-flow.[102,103] Patients with a history of at least moderate CKD who experience improvements in renal function exhibit post-LVAD survival rates comparable with those with normal preoperative renal function.[102] Concomitant CKD is a relative contraindication to LVAD placement as clinicians attempt to determine which patients experience improved renal function after implantation.[102] Patients undergoing transplantation have lower GFR compared with 20 years ago. More often, progressive renal dysfunction, however, is a sign of transition to stage 4 HF.[17] Consequently, the presence of CRS alone or in combination with other poor prognostic signs denotes a critical time to discuss end-of-life care and possibly a shift in the balance from quantity to quality of life.

END OF LIFE

Approximately 50% of HF patients die within 5 years of diagnosis.[104] Mortality is 40% to 50% per year for those with NYHA class IV symptoms.[105] Moreover, up to half of deaths from HF are sudden.[105] Survival is best predicted by the severity of disease and symptoms after treatment and not during an exacerbation.[106] Predictors of poor prognosis in CHF include renal dysfunction, liver failure, hyponatremia,[107] cardiac cachexia,[108] and an inability to be weaned off inotropes or to restore symptoms to NYHA class III despite medical optimization[101] as well as QRS widening and reduced maximal oxygen consumption, EF, heart rate, and blood pressure.[109] Kittleson and colleagues[110] demonstrated that patients unable to tolerate ACE inhibitors due to symptomatic hypotension, progressive renal dysfunction, or hyperkalemia have more severe disease and increased mortality. Furthermore, when patients are only able to tolerate extremely low doses of HF medications, the usefulness of medication continuation is unknown. Rose and colleagues[111] demonstrated that an EF less than 25%, NYHA class IV symptoms for greater than 90 days, and maximal oxygen consumption less than or equal

to 12 mL/kg/min or dependence on inotropes had a 6-month mortality of approximately 50%.

As reviewed by Goodlin in 2009,[112] through the use of appropriate medications, diet management, and other interventions, symptoms of HF can be diminished but fatigue, exertional limitations, and impaired social structure often persist. Current recommendations are to provide palliative care early in the course of HF in conjunction with therapies to prolong life.[112] Several recent reviews discuss the integration of palliative care into CHF management.[106,107,112] Some of the key points discussed in these articles include early communication and decision making about therapies, devices (implantable cardioverter defibrillator and CRT-defibrillator), goals of care, and health care proxy. Depression and patients' perceived control over their condition is tightly linked to perception of symptoms.[112] Key components of a well-rounded care plan include exercise/endurance training (eg, lower extremity strengthening and inspiratory respiratory muscle training), treatment of depression/anxiety (eg, counseling, selective serotonin reuptake inhibitors, and benzodiazepines), and management of sleep-disordered breathing (ie, continuous positive airway pressure) as well as consideration of oxygen and opioids for dyspnea.[112] The prevalence of cognitive impairment in CHF complicates recognition of worsening HF status and medication adherence.[112] Longitudinal education and psychosocial and medical support in a multidisciplinary team decrease hospitalizations, increase appropriate medication use, decrease medication errors, and improve health-related quality of life.[113] Transition toward a focus on palliation does not necessarily mean cessation of HF medications. Many patients with CHF continue taking cardiac medications indefinitely due to symptom improvement.[112] For instance, ACE inhibitors improve symptoms of HF, such as dyspnea, fatigue, orthopnea, and edema.[114] Palliative care programs have been shown to improved dyspnea, anxiety, spiritual well-being, and caregiver satisfaction and result in increased rates of death at home.[115,116] The clinical challenges of CRS will likely worsen before they get better as an aging population and HF treatment successes result in a growing number of CHF patients with end-stage cardiac and renal disease.

SUMMARY

CRS is common with 40% to 50% of stable CHF outpatients and more than 60% of those with ADHF experiencing comorbid moderate renal insufficiency. Renal insufficiency is an independent risk factor for substantial morbidity and mortality in

CHF patients. Because the pathophysiology and risk factors for CRS remain incompletely understood, the optimal acute and longitudinal management is plagued by uncertainty and common clinical dilemmas. Investigational therapies, such as adenosine antagonists, and methods for extracorporeal volume removal, such as UF and PD, may offer greater success for the future of CRS management. Palliative care and the use of a longitudinal multidisciplinary team should be instituted early in the course of CHF management to provide for the optimal balance of quantity and quality of life for all patients with CHF.

REFERENCES

1. Redfield MM, Jacobsen SJ, Burnett JC, et al. Burden of systolic and diastolic ventricular dysfunction in the community: appreciating the scope of the heart failure epidemic. JAMA 2003; 289(2):194–202.
2. Lloyd-Jones DM, Larson MG, Leip EP, et al. Lifetime risk for developing congestive heart failure: the Framingham Heart Study. Circulation 2002; 106(24):3068–72.
3. American Heart Association. 2009 Heart and stroke statistical update. Dallas (TX): American Heart Association; 2009.
4. Fonarow GC. The Acute Decompensated Heart Failure National Registry (ADHERE): opportunities to improve care of patients hospitalized with acute decompensated heart failure. Rev Cardiovasc Med 2003;4(Suppl 7):S21–30.
5. Evans F, Fakunding J. NHLBI Working Group: cardiorenal connections in heart failure and cardiovascular disease. Available at: http://www.nhlbi.nih.gov/meetings/workshops/cardiorenal-hf-hd.htm. 2004. Accessed January 10, 2010.
6. Hillege HL, Nitsch D, Pfeffer MA, et al. Renal function as a predictor of outcome in a broad spectrum of patients with heart failure. Circulation 2006; 113(5):671–8.
7. Dries DL, Exner DV, Domanski MJ, et al. The prognostic implications of renal insufficiency in asymptomatic and symptomatic patients with left ventricular systolic dysfunction. J Am Coll Cardiol 2000;35(3):681–9.
8. Schrier RW. Role of diminished renal function in cardiovascular mortality: marker or pathogenetic factor? J Am Coll Cardiol 2006;47(1):1–8.
9. Go AS, Chertow GM, Fan D, et al. Chronic kidney disease and the risks of death, cardiovascular events, and hospitalization. N Engl J Med 2004; 351(13):1296–305.
10. Manjunath G, Tighiouart H, Ibrahim H, et al. Level of kidney function as a risk factor for atherosclerotic cardiovascular outcomes in the community. J Am Coll Cardiol 2003;41(1):47–55.
11. Hillege HL, Girbes AR, de Kam PJ, et al. Renal function, neurohormonal activation, and survival in patients with chronic heart failure. Circulation 2000;102(2):203–10.
12. Shlipak MG, Smith GL, Rathore SS. Renal function, digoxin therapy, and heart failure outcomes: evidence from the digoxin intervention group trial. J Am Soc Nephrol 2004;15(8):2195–203.
13. Harnett JD, Foley RN, Kent GM, et al. Congestive heart failure in dialysis patients: prevalence, incidence, prognosis and risk factors. Kidney Int 1995;47(3):884–90.
14. Bongartz LG, Cramer MJ, Doevendans PA, et al. The severe cardiorenal syndrome: 'Guyton revisited'. Eur Heart J 2005;26(1):11–7.
15. Ronco C, Haapio M, House AA, et al. Cardiorenal syndrome. J Am Coll Cardiol 2008;52(19):1527–39.
16. Sarraf M, Masoumi A, Schrier RW. Cardiorenal syndrome in acute decompensated heart failure. Clin J Am Soc Nephrol 2009;4(12):2013–26.
17. Liang KV, Williams AW, Greene EL, et al. Acute decompensated heart failure and the cardiorenal syndrome. Crit Care Med 2008;36(Suppl 1):S75–88.
18. Krum H, Iyngkaran P, Lekawanvijit S. Pharmacologic management of the cardiorenal syndrome in heart failure. Curr Heart Fail Rep 2009;6(2):105–11.
19. McMurray JJ. Failure to practice evidence-based medicine: why do physicians not treat patients with heart failure with angiotensin-converting enzyme inhibitors? Eur Heart J 1998;19(Suppl L):L15–21.
20. Pokhrel N, Maharjan N, Dhakal B, et al. Cardiorenal syndrome: a literature review. Exp Clin Cardiol 2008;13(4):165–70.
21. Slack AJ, Wendon J. The liver and kidney in critically ill patients. Blood Purif 2009;28(2):124–34.
22. Weinfeld MS, Chertow GM, Stevenson LW. Aggravated renal dysfunction during intensive therapy for advanced chronic heart failure. Am Heart J 1999;138(2 Pt 1):285–90.
23. Cowie MR, Komajda M, Murray-Thomas T, et al. Prevalence and impact of worsening renal function in patients hospitalized with decompensated heart failure: results of the prospective outcomes study in heart failure (POSH). Eur Heart J 2006;27(10):1216–22.
24. Heywood JT, Fonarow GC, Costanzo MR, et al. High prevalence of renal dysfunction and its impact on outcome in 118,465 patients hospitalized with acute decompensated heart failure: a report from the ADHERE database. J Card Fail 2007;13(6):422–30.
25. Nohria A, Hasselblad V, Stebbins A, et al. Cardiorenal interactions: insights from the ESCAPE trial. J Am Coll Cardiol 2008;51(13):1268–74.

26. Mullens W, Abrahams Z, Francis GS, et al. Importance of venous congestion for worsening of renal function in advanced decompensated heart failure. J Am Coll Cardiol 2009;53(7):589–96.

27. Gottlieb SS, Abraham W, Butler J, et al. The prognostic importance of different definitions of worsening renal function in congestive heart failure. J Card Fail 2002;8(3):136–41.

28. Owan TE, Hodge DO, Herges RM, et al. Secular trends in renal dysfunction and outcomes in hospitalized heart failure patients. J Card Fail 2006; 12(4):257–62.

29. Krumholz HM, Chen YT, Vaccarino V, et al. Correlates and impact on outcomes of worsening renal function in patients > or =65 years of age with heart failure. Am J Cardiol 2000;85(9):1110–3.

30. Butler J, Forman DE, Abraham WT, et al. Relationship between heart failure treatment and development of worsening renal function among hospitalized patients. Am Heart J 2004;147(2):331–8.

31. Forman DE, Butler J, Wang Y, et al. Incidence, predictors at admission, and impact of worsening renal function among patients hospitalized with heart failure. J Am Coll Cardiol 2004;43(1):61–7.

32. Knight EL, Glynn RJ, McIntyre KM, et al. Predictors of decreased renal function in patients with heart failure during angiotensin-converting enzyme inhibitor therapy: results from the studies of left ventricular dysfunction (SOLVD). Am Heart J 1999;138(5 Pt 1):849–55.

33. Jose P, Skali H, Anavekar N, et al. Increase in creatinine and cardiovascular risk in patients with systolic dysfunction after myocardial infarction. J Am Soc Nephrol 2006;17(10):2886–91.

34. Smilde TD, Hillege HL, Navis G, et al. Impaired renal function in patients with ischemic and nonischemic chronic heart failure: association with neurohormonal activation and survival. Am Heart J 2004;148(1):165–72.

35. Bibbins-Domingo K, Lin F, Vittinghoff E, et al. Renal insufficiency as an independent predictor of mortality among women with heart failure. J Am Coll Cardiol 2004;44(8):1593–600.

36. Smith GL, Shlipak MG, Havranek EP, et al. Race and renal impairment in heart failure: mortality in blacks versus whites. Circulation 2005;111(10):1270–7.

37. de Silva R, Nikitin NP, Witte KK, et al. Incidence of renal dysfunction over 6 months in patients with chronic heart failure due to left ventricular systolic dysfunction: contributing factors and relationship to prognosis. Eur Heart J 2006;27(5):569–81.

38. McAlister FA, Ezekowitz J, Tonelli M, et al. Renal insufficiency and heart failure: prognostic and therapeutic implications from a prospective cohort study. Circulation 2004;109(8):1004–9.

39. Lee DS, Gona P, Vasan RS, et al. Relation of disease pathogenesis and risk factors to heart failure with preserved or reduced ejection fraction: insights from the Framingham heart study of the national heart, lung, and blood institute. Circulation 2009;119(24):3070–7.

40. Dunlay SM, Redfield MM, Weston SA, et al. Hospitalizations after heart failure diagnosis a community perspective. J Am Coll Cardiol 2009;54(18):1695–702.

41. Smith GL, Lichtman JH, Bracken MB, et al. Renal impairment and outcomes in heart failure: systematic review and meta-analysis. J Am Coll Cardiol 2006;47(10):1987–96.

42. Damman K, Navis G, Voors AA, et al. Worsening renal function and prognosis in heart failure: systematic review and meta-analysis. J Card Fail 2007;13(8):599–608.

43. Smith GL, Vaccarino V, Kosiborod M, et al. Worsening renal function: what is a clinically meaningful change in creatinine during hospitalization with heart failure? J Card Fail 2003;9(1):13–25.

44. Fonarow GC, Adams KF Jr, Abraham WT, et al. Risk stratification for in-hospital mortality in acutely decompensated heart failure: classification and regression tree analysis. JAMA 2005; 293(5):572–80.

45. Klein L, Massie BM, Leimberger JD, et al. Admission or changes in renal function during hospitalization for worsening heart failure predict postdischarge survival: results from the Outcomes of a Prospective Trial of Intravenous Milrinone for Exacerbations of Chronic Heart Failure (OPTIME-CHF). Circ Heart Fail 2008;1(1):25–33.

46. Houghton AR, Cowley AJ. Why are angiotensin converting enzyme inhibitors underutilised in the treatment of heart failure by general practitioners? Int J Cardiol 1997;59(1):7–10.

47. Ahmed A, Allman RM, DeLong JF, et al. Age-related underutilization of angiotensin-converting enzyme inhibitors in older hospitalized heart failure patients. South Med J 2002;95(7):703–10.

48. Masoudi FA, Rathore SS, Wang Y, et al. National patterns of use and effectiveness of angiotensin-converting enzyme inhibitors in older patients with heart failure and left ventricular systolic dysfunction. Circulation 2004;110(6):724–31.

49. Al-Ahmad A, Sarnak MJ, Salem DN, et al. Cause and management of heart failure in patients with chronic renal disease. Semin Nephrol 2001;21(1):3–12.

50. Al Ahmad A, Rand WM, Manjunath G, et al. Reduced kidney function and anemia as risk factors for mortality in patients with left ventricular dysfunction. J Am Coll Cardiol 2001;38(4): 955–62.

51. McClellan WM, Flanders WD, Langston RD, et al. Anemia and renal insufficiency are independent risk factors for death among patients with congestive heart failure admitted to community

hospitals: a population-based study. J Am Soc Nephrol 2002;13(7):1928–36.

52. Singh AK, Szczech L, Tang KL, et al. Correction of anemia with epoetin alfa in chronic kidney disease. N Engl J Med 2006;355:2085–98.

53. Drueke TB, Locatelli F, Clyne N, et al. Normalization of hemoglobin level in patients with chronic kidney disease and anemia. N Engl J Med 2006;355: 2071–84.

54. Goodman WG, Goldin J, Kuizon BD, et al. Coronary-artery calcification in young adults with end-stage renal disease who are undergoing dialysis. N Engl J Med 2000;342(20):1478–83.

55. Block GA, Port FK. Re-evaluation of risks associated with hyperphosphatemia and hyperparathyroidism in dialysis patients: recommendations for a change in management. Am J Kidney Dis 2000; 35(6):1226–37.

56. Sadeghi HM, Stone GW, Grines CL, et al. Impact of renal insufficiency in patients undergoing primary angioplasty for acute myocardial infarction. Circulation 2003;108(22):2769–75.

57. Russo D, Palmiero G, De Blasio AP, et al. Coronary artery calcification in patients with CRF not undergoing dialysis. Am J Kidney Dis 2004;44: 1024–30.

58. Ketteler M, Schlieper G, Floege J. Calcification and cardiovascular health: new insights into an old phenomenon. Hypertension 2006;47: 1027–34.

59. Schiffrin EL, Lipman ML, Mann JF. Chronic kidney disease: effects on the cardiovascular system. Circulation 2007;116:85–97.

60. Shlipak MG, Fried LF, Crump C, et al. Elevations of inflammatory and procoagulant biomarkers in elderly persons with renal insufficiency. Circulation 2003;107(1):87–92.

61. Boushey CJ, Beresford SA, Omenn GS, et al. A quantitative assessment of plasma homocysteine as a risk factor for vascular disease. Probable benefits of increasing folic acid intakes. JAMA 1995;274(13):1049–57.

62. Gerstein HC, Mann JF, Yi Q, et al. Albuminuria and risk of cardiovascular events, death, and heart failure in diabetic and nondiabetic individuals. JAMA 2001;286(4):421–6.

63. Taki K, Tsuruta Y, Niwa T. Indoxyl sulfate and atherosclerotic risk factors in hemodialysis patients. Am J Nephrol 2007;27(1):30–5.

64. Lee WH, Packer M. Prognostic importance of serum sodium concentration and its modification by converting-enzyme inhibition in patients with severe chronic heart failure. Circulation 1986; 73(2):257–67.

65. Leier CV, Dei Cas L, Metra M. Clinical relevance and management of the major electrolyte abnormalities in congestive heart failure: hyponatremia,

hypokalemia, and hypomagnesemia. Am Heart J 1994;128(3):564–74.

66. Salvador DR, Rey NR, Ramos GC, et al. Continuous infusion versus bolus injection of loop diuretics in congestive heart failure. Cochrane Database Syst Rev 2005;(3):CD003178.

67. Shlipak MG. Pharmacotherapy for heart failure in patients with renal insufficiency. Ann Intern Med 2003;138(11):917–24.

68. Gattis WA, O'Connor CM, Leimberger JD, et al. Clinical outcomes in patients on beta-blocker therapy admitted with worsening chronic heart failure. Am J Cardiol 2003;91(2):169–74. OPTIME.

69. Metra M, Torp-Pedersen C, Cleland JG, et al. Should beta-blocker therapy be reduced or withdrawn after an episode of decompensated heart failure? Results from COMET. Eur J Heart Fail 2007;9(9):901–9.

70. Butler J, Young JB, Abraham WT, et al. Beta-blocker use and outcomes among hospitalized heart failure patients. J Am Coll Cardiol 2006; 47(12):2462–9.

71. Fonarow GC, Abraham WT, Albert NM, et al. Influence of beta-blocker continuation or withdrawal on outcomes in patients hospitalized with heart failure: findings from the OPTIMIZE-HF program. J Am Coll Cardiol 2008;52(3):190–9.

72. Butler J, Arbogast PG, BeLue R, et al. Outpatient adherence to beta-blocker therapy after acute myocardial infarction. J Am Coll Cardiol 2002; 40(9):1589–95.

73. Sackner-Bernstein JD, Skopicki HA, Aaronson KD. Risk of worsening renal function with nesiritide in patients with acutely decompensated heart failure. Circulation 2005;111(12):1487–91.

74. Arora RR, Venkatesh PK, Molnar J. Short and long-term mortality with nesiritide. Am Heart J 2006; 152(6):1084–90.

75. ASCEND-HF. Double-blind, placebo-controlled, multicenter acute study of clinical effectiveness of nesiritide in subjects with decompensated heart failure. Available at: http://clinicaltrials.gov/ct2/show/NCT00475852. Accessed January 10, 2010.

76. Schrier RW, Gross P, Gheorghiade M, et al. Tolvaptan, a selective oral vasopressin V2-receptor antagonist, for hyponatremia. N Engl J Med 2006; 355(20):2099–112.

77. Gheorghiade M, Niazi I, Ouyang J, et al. Vasopressin V2-receptor blockade with tolvaptan in patients with chronic heart failure: results from a double-blind, randomized trial. Circulation 2003; 107(21):2690–6.

78. Gheorghiade M, Gattis WA, O'Connor CM, et al. Effects of tolvaptan, a vasopressin antagonist, in patients hospitalized with worsening heart failure: a randomized controlled trial. JAMA 2004; 291(16):1963–71.

79. Cotter G, Dittrich HC, Weatherley BD, et al. The PROTECT pilot study: a randomized, placebo-controlled, dose-finding study of the adenosine A1 receptor antagonist rolofylline in patients with acute heart failure and renal impairment. J Card Fail 2008;14(8):631–40.

80. Kazory A, Ross EA. Contemporary trends in the pharmacological and extracorporeal management of heart failure: a nephrologic perspective. Circulation 2008;117(7):975–83.

81. Jessup M, Costanzo MR. The cardiorenal syndrome: do we need a change of strategy or a change of tactics? J Am Coll Cardiol 2009;53(7):597–9.

82. Khalifeh N, Vychytil A, Hörl WH. The role of peritoneal dialysis in the management of treatment-resistant congestive heart failure: a European perspective. Kidney Int Suppl 2006;103:S72–5.

83. Liang KV, Hiniker AR, Williams AW, et al. Use of a novel ultrafiltration device as a treatment strategy for diuretic resistant, refractory heart failure: initial clinical experience in a single center. J Card Fail 2006;12(9):707–14.

84. Costanzo MR, Guglin ME, Saltzberg MT, et al. Ultrafiltration versus intravenous diuretics for patients hospitalized for acute decompensated heart failure. J Am Coll Cardiol 2007;49(6):675–83.

85. Krishnan A, Oreopoulos DG. Peritoneal dialysis in congestive heart failure. Adv Perit Dial 2007;23:82–9.

86. Gotloib L, Fudin R, Yakubovich M, et al. Peritoneal dialysis in refractory end-stage congestive heart failure: a challenge facing a no-win situation. Nephrol Dial Transplant 2005;20(Suppl 7):vii32–6.

87. Stack AG, Molony DA, Rahman NS, et al. Impact of dialysis modality on survival of new ESRD patients with congestive heart failure in the United States. Kidney Int 2003;64(3):1071–9.

88. Couchoud C, Stengel B, Landais P, et al. The renal epidemiology and information network (REIN): a new registry for end-stage renal disease in France. Nephrol Dial Transplant 2006;21:411–8.

89. Kirchgessner J, Pera-Chang M, Klinkner G, et al. Satisfaction with care in peritoneal dialysis patients. Kidney Int 2006;70:1325–31.

90. Frimat L, Durand PY, Loos-Avay C, et al. Impact of first dialysis modality on outcome of patients contraindicated for kidney transplant. Perit Dial Int 2006;26:231–9.

91. Gheorghiade M, Filippatos G. Reassessing treatment of acute heart failure syndromes: the ADHERE registry. Eur Heart J 2005;7(Suppl B):B13–9.

92. Roy P, Bouchard J, Amyot R, et al. Prescription patterns of pharmacological agents for left ventricular systolic dysfunction among hemodialysis patients. Am J Kidney Dis 2006;48(4):645–51.

93. Ruggenenti P, Perna A, Remuzzi G. ACE inhibitors to prevent end-stage renal disease: when to start and why possibly never to stop: a post hoc analysis of the REIN trial results. Ramipril efficacy in nephropathy. J Am Soc Nephrol 2001;12(12):2832–7.

94. Bakris GL, Weir MR. Angiotensin-converting enzyme inhibitorassociated elevations in serum creatinine: is this a cause for concern? Arch Intern Med 2000;160:685–93.

95. Effects of enalapril on mortality in severe congestive heart failure. Results of the Cooperative North Scandinavian Enalapril Survival Study (CONSENSUS). The CONSENSUS Trial Study Group. N Engl J Med 1987;316(23):1429–35.

96. Ljungman S, Kjekshus J, Swedberg K. Renal function in severe congestive heart failure during treatment with enalapril (the Cooperative North Scandinavian Enalapril Survival Study [CONSENSUS] Trial). Am J Cardiol 1992;70(4):479–87.

97. MacDowall P, Kalra PA, O'Donoghue DJ, et al. Risk of morbidity from renovascular disease in elderly patients with congestive cardiac failure. Lancet 1998;352(9121):13–6.

98. Shlipak MG, Browner WS, Noguchi H, et al. Comparison of the effects of angiotensin converting-enzyme inhibitors and beta blockers on survival in elderly patients with reduced left ventricular function after myocardial infarction. Am J Med 2001;110(6):425–33.

99. Pitt B, Zannad F, Remme WJ, et al. The effect of spironolactone on morbidity and mortality in patients with severe heart failure. Randomized Aldactone Evaluation Study Investigators. N Engl J Med 1999;341(10):709–17.

100. The effect of digoxin on mortality and morbidity in patients with heart failure. The Digitalis Investigation Group. N Engl J Med 1997;336(8):525–33.

101. Wilson SR, Mudge GH Jr, Stewart GC, et al. Evaluation for a ventricular assist device: selecting the appropriate candidate. Circulation 2009;119(16):2225–32.

102. Sandner SE, Zimpfer D, Zrunek P, et al. Renal function and outcome after continuous flow left ventricular assist device implantation. Ann Thorac Surg 2009;87(4):1072–8.

103. Kamdar F, Boyle A, Liao K, et al. Effects of centrifugal, axial, and pulsatile left ventricular assist device support on end-organ function in heart failure patients. J Heart Lung Transplant 2009;28(4):352–9.

104. Heart disease and stroke statistics—2004 update. Dallas (TX): American Heart Association; 2000.

105. Stevenson WG, Stevenson LW. Prevention of sudden death in heart failure. J Cardiovasc Electrophysiol 2001;12(1):112–4.

106. Pantilat SZ, Steimle AE. Palliative care for patients with heart failure. JAMA 2004;291(20):2476–82.

107. Hauptman PJ, Havranek EP. Integrating palliative care into heart failure care. Arch Intern Med 2005;165(4):374–8.

108. Anker SD, Chua TP, Ponikowski P, et al. Hormonal changes and catabolic/anabolic imbalance in chronic heart failure and their importance for cardiac cachexia. Circulation 1997;96(2):526–34.

109. Aaronson KD, Schwartz JS, Chen TM, et al. Development and prospective validation of a clinical index to predict survival in ambulatory patients referred for cardiac transplant evaluation. Circulation 1997;95(12):2660–7.

110. Kittleson M, Hurwitz S, Shah MR, et al. Development of circulatory-renal limitations to angiotensin-converting enzyme inhibitors identifies patients with severe heart failure and early mortality. J Am Coll Cardiol 2003;41(11):2029–35.

111. Rose EA, Gelijns AC, Moskowitz AJ, et al. Long-term mechanical left ventricular assistance for end-stage heart failure. N Engl J Med 2001; 345(20):1435–43.

112. Goodlin SJ. Palliative care in congestive heart failure. J Am Coll Cardiol 2009;54(5):386–96.

113. Phillips CO, Wright SM, Kern DE, et al. Comprehensive discharge planning with postdischarge support for older patients with congestive heart failure: a meta-analysis. JAMA 2004;291(11):1358–67.

114. A placebo-controlled trial of captopril in refractory chronic congestive heart failure. Captopril Multicenter Research Group. J Am Coll Cardiol 1983; 2(4):755–63.

115. Rabow MW, Dibble SL, Pantilat SZ, et al. The comprehensive care team: a controlled trial of outpatient palliative medicine consultation. Arch Intern Med 2004;164(1):83–91.

116. Brumley R, Enguidanos S, Jamison P, et al. Increased satisfaction with care and lower costs: results of a randomized trial of in-home palliative care. J Am Geriatr Soc 2007;55(7):993–1000.

Anemia in Chronic Kidney Disease: New Advances

Tejas V. Patel, MD, Ajay K. Singh, MB, FRCP(UK)*

KEYWORDS

- Anemia • Chronic kidney disease
- Cardiovascular disease • Hepcidin • Iron
- Ferumoxytol • Erythropoietin

Anemia is a common complication of chronic kidney disease (CKD) and is primarily caused by deficiency of erythropoietin (EPO) and iron, patients who are anemic have higher complication rates, Including increased number of hospitalizations, left ventricular hypertrophy, and death.[1] By the time patients with CKD are on dialysis (CKD-D), more than 70% will require treatment for anemia. Our understanding of the pathophysiology of anemia in CKD has significantly advanced in the past decade, more so in the past 3 years. The authors divided this article into four sections. The first section concentrates on iron homeostasis and iron treatment. The second section evaluates target hemoglobin (Hgb) levels with erythropoiesis-stimulating agents (ESA). The third section explores the mechanism of higher mortality with anemia treatment and the last section focuses on newer molecules used to treat anemia in CKD.

ADVANCES IN IRON HOMEOSTASIS

Despite an abundance of iron available in nature, its metabolism is tightly regulated. For instance, although the total iron content in the body is 40 to 50 mg/kg, there is only 70 mg of bio-available iron. Further, the amount of iron lost generally equals the amount of iron absorbed from the gastrointestinal tract, about 1 to 2 mg daily.

Because free ferrous is a potent catalyst, iron remains predominantly sequestered by transferrin (transport protein); transferrin receptor (present on the surface of erythroid precursors); and ferritin (to store iron in the reticulo-endothelial system).[2,3] Serum transferrin binds one to two Fe^{3+} atoms and iron-bound transferrin circulates freely in the serum. Excess intracellular iron is stored in ferritin, which can store up to 5000 iron atoms inside its shell.[4] **Fig. 1** depicts the distribution of iron in adults.

During the past decade, there have been tremendous advances in our understanding of iron physiology in normal and disease states, in particular kidney disease. Two independent research teams coincidentally discovered a peptide associated with inflammation known as liver expressed antimicrobial protein, later termed hepcidin, as it was produced by the liver and had bactericidal properties. Excess production of hepcidin was also seen in iron overload.[5] A group from Boston subsequently reported that subjects with liver tumors who also had resistant iron-deficiency anemia were cured of anemia upon tumor removal. These subjects were found to produce large quantities of hepcidin.[6] These series of events catapulted the field of molecular basis of iron-deficiency anemia, especially in patients with "anemia of chronic disease."[7]

Conflict of Interest: Dr Patel reports no conflicts of interest. Dr Singh discloses receiving consulting fees from Johnson & Johnson and Watson, lecture fees from Johnson & Johnson, Amgen, and Watson, and grant support from Johnson & Johnson, Amgen, Roche, AMAG Pharmaceuticals, and Watson.

Renal Division, Brigham and Women's Hospital, 75 Francis Street, Boston, MA 02115, USA

* Corresponding author.

E-mail address: asingh@rics.bwh.harvard.edu

Heart Failure Clin 6 (2010) 347–357
doi:10.1016/j.hfc.2010.02.001
1551-7136/10/$ – see front matter © 2010 Published by Elsevier Inc.

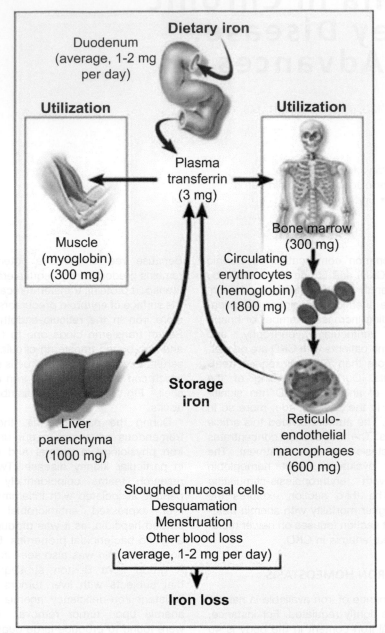

Fig. 1. Distribution of iron in adults. In the balanced state, 1 to 2 mg of iron enters and leaves the body each day. Dietary iron is absorbed by duodenal enterocytes. It circulates in plasma bound to transferrin. Most of the iron in the body is incorporated into hemoglobin in erythroid precursors and mature red cells. Approximately 10% to 15% is present in muscle fibers (in myoglobin) and other tissues (in enzymes and cytochromes). Iron is stored in parenchymal cells of the liver and reticuloendothelial macrophages. These macrophages provide most of the usable iron by degrading hemoglobin in senescent erythrocytes and reloading ferric iron onto transferrin for delivery to cells (*From* Andrews N. Disorders of iron metabolism. N Engl J Med 1999;341:1986; with permission.)

The Role of the Intestine and Liver in Iron Homeostasis

Iron is predominantly absorbed in the proximal duodenum. Non-heme iron, ferric (Fe^{3+}), needs to be reduced to ferrous (Fe^{2+}) by a luminal ferric reductase. Subsequently, ferrous iron enters the enterocyte carried by an iron transporter, divalent metal transporter 1 (DMT1). Once in the cell, the iron may stay within the enterocyte or get transported outside the cell via a basolateral iron transporter, ferroportin. The binding of hepcidin, a 25-amino acid protein, to the cell surface ferroportin triggers phosphorylation and eventual internalization and degradation of the transporter.[8] Inactivation of ferroportin results in inhibition of iron transport across the basolateral membrane of enterocytes, which translates into iron deficiency. On the other hand, inactivation of hepcidin results in unopposed expression of ferroportin and thus iron overload. Because iron cannot be excreted by the kidney, the hepcidin-ferroportin axis acts as a central regulator of iron homeostasis in the body. Similarly, high hepcidin levels in macrophages blocks iron transport into the circulation. Factors that suppress hepcidin are hypoxia or hypoxia-inducible factor (HIF); growth differentiation factor-15; and erythropoiesis. In contrast, inflammatory interleukins, such as IL-6 and iron treatment, stimulate hepcidin.[9] A cartoon depicting hepcidin regulating iron is illustrated in **Fig. 2**.

The exact mechanism of activation of hepcidin is still under intense investigation. The most important pathway seems to be through the bone morphogenic protein (BMP). BMP binds to the cell surface receptor (mainly hemojuvelin) and activates SMAD (proteins that modulate transforming growth factor beta) signaling thereby promoting hepcidin gene expression.[10] The data is supported by reports of iron overload in patients with hemojuvelin mutation.[11]

Role of Kidney in Iron Homeostasis

The role of kidney in iron homeostasis has evolved over the past decade. It is now known that transferrin is an essential growth factor for the development of kidneys, and differentiation of tubule and filtering and retrieval of transferrin from the filtrate provides iron for tubular metabolism.[12] Series of in vitro and in vivo experiments have uncovered the role of kidneys in regulating transferrin and ferritin by ubiquitously present cytosolic proteins: iron regulatory proteins (IRP) 1 and 2.[4] IRP2 deficiency results in microcytic anemia, high ferritin and several fold increase in erythropoietin levels.[13]

In the presence of normal oxygen tension, iron (Fe^{2+})-dependent prolyl hydroxylases are active in hydroxylating HIF 1α and 2α. Hydroxylated HIF gets degraded by Von Hippel-Lindau (VHL) complex, an onco-suppressor. Thus in iron deficiency, HIF levels may increase, which may enhance erythropoietin secretion by renal fibroblast. Alternatively, VHL mutation increases HIF levels, which in turn would increase iron availability.[14]

In summary, role of kidney in iron regulation is increasingly being recognized but more research is needed to better understand its role in iron homeostasis.

Clinical Studies Evaluating Hepcidin in Chronic Kidney Disease

Because of the small size and evolutionary conservation of hepcidin, sensitive immunoassays have been a challenge. Use of hepcidin precursor, serum pro-hepcidin has not been informative of the iron physiology. Urinary hepcidin studies in humans have had good correlation with the serum hepcidin.[15] Only recently, because of availability

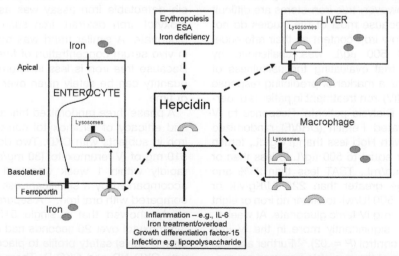

Fig. 2. Role of hepcidin in iron homeostasis. The activity of hepcidin is depicted showing ferroportin as a target on enterocytes and macrophages. Hepcidin binds to ferroportin triggering its internalization and lysosomal degradation. Factors influencing hepcidin expression are also outlined. Horseshoe-shape represents hepcidin; the rectangle represents ferroportin. Solid arrow enhances activity; broken arrow suppresses activity of hepcidin.

of ELISA and mass spectrometry-based assays for hepcidin, clinical studies have started to evaluate the serum hepcidin levels in subjects with kidney disease. Valenti and colleagues published the first human study in subjects with CKD evaluating serum hepcidin levels. Serum from 65 subjects with hemodialysis (HD) and 57 healthy controls was evaluated for hepcidin-25. Hepcidin-25 was higher in subjects with HD and correlated positively with ferritin and C-reactive protein and negatively with serum iron. Further, HFE mutation modulated hepcidin levels in subjects with HD.[16] Another study reported hepcidin correlated well with ferritin and soluble transferrin receptor ($R^2 = 0.78$) in non-dialysis subjects with CKD (CKD-ND).[9] Hepcidin-25 is filtered and reabsorbed in the proximal tubule, making urinary hepcidin an attractive biomarker of renal function.[17] It is important to point out that there is a tremendous variation among different hepcidin assays and the authors would urge caution when interpreting the findings.[18]

ADVANCES IN THE MANAGEMENT OF IRON DEFICIENCY

The National Kidney Foundation/Disease Outcome Quality Initiative (K/DOQI) guideline states that iron stores are adequate if serum ferritin is greater than 100 µg/L in CKD-ND and greater than 200 µg/L in patients who have CKD-D with transferrin saturation (TSAT) greater than 20%.[19] Epidemiologic studies have found that sensitivity of serum ferritin in excluding iron deficiency anemia is 98% to 100% at levels greater than 500 µg/L.[20] However, true iron stores are difficult to ascertain because most of the studies do not use bone marrow iron content as their reference. The cutoff of 500 µg/L was challenged by a randomized trial evaluating the usefulness of serum ferritin as a marker of predicting response to intravenous (IV) iron treatment in patients undergoing dialysis. Dialysis patients' Response to IV Iron with Elevated Ferritin (DRIVE) randomized 134 subjects with Hgb less than 11 g/dL, ferritin greater than or equal to 500 µg/L to less than or equal to 1200µg/mL, TSAT less than 25% and epoetin dosage greater than 225 IU/Kg/wk or greater than 22,500 IU/wk to either no iron or eight sessions of 125 mg IV ferric gluconate. At week 6, Hgb increased significantly more in the IV iron group than the control ($P = .02$).[21] Further analysis found that none of the available iron markers predicted response to IV iron: ferritin, reticulocytes Hgb content, soluble transferrin receptor, or transferrin saturation.[22] This study underscores the need for a reliable noninvasive clinical marker for iron deficiency in patients with CKD.

Intravenous iron products have been the treatment of choice for iron deficiency in patients with advanced CKD and end-stage renal disease.[23] A high incidence of allergic reactions[24] to the initial IV iron preparation of iron dextran (INFed, Watson Pharmaceuticals, Corona, CA and DexFerrum, American Regent Inc, Shirley, NY, USA) resulted in its infrequent use. Low-molecular weight iron dextran may be better tolerated.[25] Newer IV iron preparations, such as sodium ferric gluconate (Ferrlecit, Watson Pharmaceuticals Inc, Corona, CA, USA) and iron sucrose (Venofer, American Regent Inc, Shirley, NY, USA), may have lower incidences of allergic reaction, but they need to be administered in small doses and as a slow push or infusion because greater doses or faster rates of administration are associated with serious adverse events.[26,27] Thus, administration of 1g of iron can take many sessions.

The most recent addition, ferumoxytol (Feraheme, AMAG Pharmaceuticals Inc, Lexington, MA, USA), a semisynthetic, carbohydrate-coated superparamagnetic iron oxide nanoparticle was recently approved by the US Food and Drug Administration (FDA) to treat iron-deficiency anemia in CKD.[28] It contains less free iron than other IV iron preparations. In vivo and in vitro comparing low-molecular iron dextran, iron sucrose, and iron ferric gluconate showed ferumoxytol being least ultrafiltrable and dialyzable. Incubation of intravenous iron preparations in rat or pooled human sera demonstrated minimal free iron release with ferumoxytol. The order of catalytic iron release as detected by the bleomycin detectable iron assay was as follows: ferumoxytol, iron dextran, iron sucrose, and ferric gluconate. A similar trend was observed for the in vivo serum concentration of free iron in rats.[29] Because free iron is less in ferumoxytol, a large quantity can be safely given over a short period of time.

A phase three randomized trial assessed safety and efficacy of ferumoxytol compared with oral iron in subjects with CKD. Two dosages each of 510 mg of IV ferumoxytol (30 mg/s) administered rapidly within 1 week was well tolerated and accompanied by a significant rise in hemoglobin compared with oral iron.[30] A separate phase three study showed that a single 510 mg dose of ferumoxytol over 20 seconds had a similar short-term (7 days) safety profile to placebo in subjects with CKD-ND and CKD-D. There was no significant decrease in blood pressure after administration of the active agent,[31] a commonly feared side effect of IV iron administration. However, long-term safety of any of the iron compounds remains to be evaluated in a randomized trial.

Finally, harnessing treatment agents from our understanding of hepcidin and related molecules will be an important step forward in the management of iron deficiency anemia. For instance, suppressing hepcidin or modulating one of its gene promoters (eg, hemojuvelin) may enhance iron absorption and complement current iron treatments.[32]

EVOLVING HEMOGLOBIN TARGET LEVEL

Recombinant EPO (rEPO) has been successfully used to treat anemia in patients with CKD for almost 20 years. The US FDA approved the use of rEPO on the basis of a rise in hematocrit and a reduction in the need for blood transfusions in a small number of patients undergoing hemodialysis over a 3-week period.[33] Because of changes in reimbursement policies by Medicare, the use of epoetin dramatically increased with a resultant increase in hemoglobin.[34] Epidemiologic studies reported that treatment of anemia with rEPO improved not only surrogate markers, such as left ventricular hypertrophy and quality of life, but also survival.[35,36] However, randomized trials addressing mortality were lacking. The results of randomized trials in subjects with CKD-D and CKD-ND have been disappointing. The Normal Hematocrit Study from more than a decade ago randomized 1233 subjects with prevalent hemodialysis with clinical evidence of congestive heart failure or ischemic heart disease to achieve and maintain a hematocrit of 42% by increasing epoetin dose versus maintaining a hematocrit of 30% throughout the study by adjusting the epoetin dose. After 29 months, the study was halted as there was a trend for increased death in the normal-hematocrit group compared with the low-hematocrit group (risk 1.3, CI 0.9 to 1.9).[37]

In November 2006, two independent, randomized trials reported similar concerning findings in subjects with CKD-ND. The Correction of Hemoglobin and Outcomes in Renal Insufficiency (CHOIR, http://ClinicalTrials.gov number, NCT00211120) trial studied 1432 subjects with CKD in an open-label randomized trial: 715 assigned to receive epoetin alfa targeted to achieve a Hgb level of 13.5 g/dL and 717 targeted to achieve a Hgb of 11.3 g/dL. After following for a median of 16 months, the primary end point of composite of death; myocardial infarction; hospitalization for congestive heart failure (without renal replacement therapy); and stroke occurred more frequently in the high-Hgb group compared with the low-Hgb group (125 events vs 97 events,

hazard ratio [HR] 1.34; 95% CI 1.03 to 1.74, P = .03). Further, there was no difference in improvements in quality of life between the groups.[38] A parallel study, Cardiovascular Risk Reduction by Early Anemia Treatment with Epoetin Beta (CREATE trial, http://ClinicalTrials.gov number, NCT00321919) assigned 603 subjects to either a target Hgb range of 13 to15 g/dL or a target Hgb range of 10.5 to 11.5 g/dL. During the 3 years of follow-up, primary end point of a composite of cardiovascular events was similar in both groups (58 events in high-Hgb vs 47 events in low-Hgb group, hazard ratio, P = .20). There was no difference in left ventricular mass index and glomerular filtration rate decline. However, dialysis was required in more subjects in the high-Hgb group (P = .03). Improvement in quality of life was significantly better in the high-Hgb group.[39] Although some have been critical of the these trials,[40] collectively these trials have demonstrated increased risk for ESA therapy in correcting CKD anemia. A subsequent meta-analysis also found 16% higher mortality in subjects targeted to higher Hgb.[41] The 2007 Kidney Disease Outcomes Quality Initiative (K/DOQI) guidelines update revised their recommendation to a target Hgb between 11 g/dL to 12 g/dL and not to overshoot Hgb above 13 g/dL.[19] More recently, the Trial to Reduce cardiovascular Events with Aranesp Therapy[42] (TREAT, http://ClinicalTrials.gov number, NCT00093015) was published. It is the largest trial in nephrology that confirms the adverse outcomes in subjects targeted to high-hgb. However, unlike previous studies, TREAT compared active agent (darbepoietin) to a placebo. The study randomized more than 4000 subjects with CKD-ND with type 2 diabetes mellitus to either treatment with darbepoietin alfa to achieve Hgb approximately 13 g/dL or placebo with rescue darbepoietin alfa when the hemoglobin level was less than 9.0 g/dL. After a median follow-up of 29.1 months per subject, though there was no difference in total deaths, CV events, dialysis requirement, or hospitalizations, pre-specified outcome of fatal or non-fatal stroke was significantly higher in the active arm (101 in darbepoietin vs 53 in placebo, HR 1.92, P<.001). Also, there was higher incidence of arterial and venous thromboembolism in the active group (P = .02) and death from cancer in patients with a history of malignancy. A trend for higher incidence of hypertension was also observed (P = .07). There was only a modest improvement in subject-reported fatigue in the darbepoietin alfa group as compared with placebo. As expected the number of blood transfusions was higher in the placebo arm. The authors cautioned against using the drug as the risks outweighed the potential benefits.[42] The findings of this study confirm that there is no mortality or cardiovascular benefit from ESA in patients who are anemic with CKD but a consistent finding of higher adverse outcomes.

In summary, the management of anemia in CKD-ND has undergone significant revision in the past 3 years. Collectively, these trials point to hemoglobin being a flawed intermediate clinical outcome (ie, correcting the hemoglobin is not associated with improved hard endpoints, such as mortality or cardiovascular complications). These trials also raise the question of whether ESA exposure rather than a higher hemoglobin should be implicated.

MECHANISM OF HIGHER ADVERSE EVENTS IN PATIENTS WHO ARE ANEMIC WITH CHRONIC KIDNEY DISEASE TREATED WITH ERYTHROPOIESIS-STIMULATING AGENTS AND IRON

Multiple mechanisms have been proposed to explain the higher mortality seen in patients with CKD treated with iron and ESA.[43] Higher Hgb alone and associated blood volume expansion may stress the cardiovascular system. Recently, a post-hoc study of the CHOIR trial reported that analyses at 4 months and 9 months showed high-dose epoetin-alpha was associated with a significant increased hazard of primary end point (death, myocardial infarction, congestive heart failure, or stroke) in subjects who did not achieve the targeted Hgb and there was no increased risk associated with achieving higher Hgb.[44]

Therefore, failure to achieve the targeted Hgb in the setting of exposure to high epoetin dose may increase mortality. The underlying mechanism is an area of active investigation. The authors' cross-sectional data in 100 subjects with CKD-ND showed significantly higher levels of tumor necrosis factor α (TNFα) and trend for higher levels of IL-6 and IL-8 in subjects receiving ESA compared with subjects not receiving ESA.[45] Platelet activation has been proposed as a mechanism for higher CVD events in patients exposed to ESA. In a separate analysis in subjects with CKD-ND, exposure to ESA was associated with higher levels of soluble P-selectin, a marker of platelet activation.[46] Longitudinal studies are needed to confirm the findings from these cross-sectional trials. In subjects undergoing dialysis, modest doses of EPO (4000 units and 8000 units) showed increased oxidative stress markers of plasma malondialdehyde and iso-PGF2 and reduction in antioxidant capacity (total antioxidant activity and nitrite/nitrate concentration).[47] Thus, surrogate markers of adverse outcome have been linked to ESA, though the significance of each remains to be determined.

Increased blood pressure is the most prominent side effect when treating patients with ESA.[48] The potential mechanisms for ESA-induced hypertension have been discussed in great length elsewhere.[49] To avoid the hypertensive effects of ESA, Lee and colleagues reported the effects of EPO-binding protein (bp) and anti-EPO antibodies in Dawley-Sprague rats. They showed that treatment of EPO with EPO-bp or anti-EPO–bp maintained blood pressure at similar levels as saline treatment without affecting hematocrit or blood volume.[50] Thus, it is possible to avoid hypertensive effects of EPO without compromising its ability to correct anemia. Further work is needed to translate this basic scientific finding into clinically meaningful therapeutic modality.

Progression of cancer has emerged as one of the most concerning findings linked to ESA.[51] It is not yet known if this effect results from enhanced angiogenesis via vascular endothelial growth factor (VEGF) or an independent pathway.[52] Further, tumor cells express EPO receptors.[53] The TREAT trial had statistically significant higher death from cancer in subjects with a history of solid malignancy. Therefore, any future anemia treatment would need to keep this unintended side effect in mind.

The increase in incidence of stroke in TREAT and higher cardiovascular events in CHOIR may be related to differential effects of the type of ESA used. Investigators from Britain examined the effect of darbepoietin and epoetin beta on mice retina. They reported that darbepoietin showed more potent release of TNFα and VEGF compared with epoetin beta.[54] Clearly, further work needs to be performed, but this finding may in part explain the differences in adverse effects between the different molecules.

Intravenous iron treatment may play a role in adverse outcomes as free iron has been implicated to oxidant stress, higher risk for infection and cardiovascular risk.[55] There is evidence that even newer IV iron preparations are proinflammatory and cause oxidative stress and even proteinuria.[56] The mechanism of proteinuria is thought to be from transient cytokine release. However, high molecular weight of the iron preparation may play a role. Iron also causes direct tubular damage in cell culture.[57,58] Thus, it has been hypothesized that IV iron treatment may be related to higher mortality associated with targeting higher Hgb.[43] The Normal Hematocrit Study and CHOIR had higher requirement of IV iron in subjects targeted to higher Hgb. However, in the TREAT study, the placebo arm had significantly higher IV iron use. It seems that iron is probably not the main culprit.

Patient characteristics, such as diabetes, congestive heart failure, and cardiovascular disease, may play a role in influencing outcomes. A post-hoc analysis of CHOIR could not uncover any subject sub-population at higher risk for adverse outcomes.[59] Hopefully post-hoc analysis of TREAT or subject-level meta-analysis may give more information.

In summary, although the authors have explored multiple mechanisms that may partially explain the higher mortality linked to ESA, further work needs to be done to elucidate relative importance of these mechanisms to enable better clinical management. **Fig. 3** summarizes the section.

NEWER MOLECULES FOR TREATING ANEMIA
Erythropoietin Receptor Activator

Epoetin alfa, a glycoprotein of 165-amino acids has a half-life of 6 to 8 hours when given intravenously and 18 to 24 hours when given subcutaneously. Thus, it needs to be administered up to three times a week in patients undergoing dialysis and weekly in patients with CKD-ND. Longer-acting, erythropoiesis-stimulating agents have been created by adding heavy glycoprotein chain to the EPO molecule. Darbepoietin alfa, produced by site-directed mutagenesis, has two N-terminal linked oligosaccharide chains and has significantly longer half-life: 25 hours by intravenous and 48 hours by subcutaneous administration, allowing for less frequent administration (every 2 weeks

subcutaneously in patients with CKD-ND).[60] A large methoxy-polyethylene glycol chain to EPO significantly increases the half-life; Continuous Erythropoietin Receptor Activator (CERA) increases half-life up to 130 hours, which enables administration every 2 to 4 weeks. The drug has less affinity for the EPO receptor but a higher stability compared with EPO. However, because of legal issues over patent infringement, the marketing of this molecule has been banned in the United States.[61]

Bio-Similars

Several small, unrelated peptides induce the EPO receptor. One such peptide, Hematide (Affymax Inc., Palo Alto, CA), is a pegylated synthetic dimeric peptide ESA that increased the reticulocyte count in a Phase one study.[62] A phase two study showed that a monthly administration had a predictable response with no significant influence of age, gender, race, and underlying CKD etiology.[63] Other peptides (HX575, Binocrit, and epoetin zeta) have been approved by the European Medicine Agency.[64] The potential advantages are lower immunogenicity, lack of anti-EPO antibodies cross reacting, and less expensive manufacturing process.[65,66] However, standardized manufacturing process of these peptides is lacking.

GATA Inhibitors

Erythropoietin gene expression is under the control of HIF1, and is negatively regulated by GATA, a family of transcription factors that bind

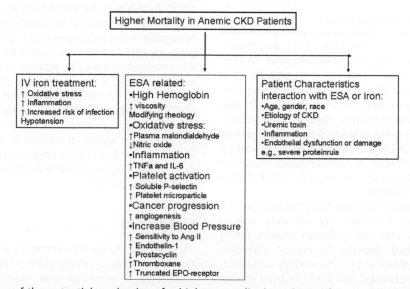

Fig. 3. Summary of the potential mechanisms for higher mortality in patients who are anemic and have CKD.

to the sequence GATA. Interleukin 1β and TNFα increase the binding activity of GATA and inhibit EPO promoter activity. In an elegant study by Nakano and colleagues, in vitro and in vivo mouse study reported anemia induced by IL-1β and TNFα was ameliorated by oral administration of K-11,706, a GATA-2 inhibitor. The Hgb, EPO levels, reticulocytes, and colony forming units-erythroid increased.[67]

Hypoxia-Inducible Factor Stabilizers

As discussed in the earlier section, under normal oxygen tension, EPO gene expression is suppressed by inhibition of HIF, which in turn is mediated by prolyl hydroxylases. Prolyl hydroxylase inhibitors termed HIF stabilizers are molecules that promote expression of endogenous EPO by modulating iron (eg, elevated Dcytb, DMT1, transferrin and its receptor, and decreased hepcidin) and 2-oxogluatarate availability.[68] In animal studies of fifth-sixth nephrectomy rats, compared with EPO, HIF stabilizers (FG-2216 and FG-4592, Fibrogen Inc, San Francisco, CA) increased hemoglobin without exacerbating hypertension.[69] Phase two studies of orally administered compound have shown increases in EPO and reticulocyte count and improved iron use. However, these agents tend to upregulate other HIF sensitive genes, namely VEGF, which has theoretical concern of tumor growth. Most recently, a phase one study of HIF-PH stabilizer AKB-6548, a single dose of orally active drug, showed promising results in 48 healthy volunteers. According to a press release, there was no significant change in VEGF levels.[70]

Other Treatment Modalities

Hemopoietic cell phosphatase (HCP), an intracellular protein that is a negative regulator of EPO receptor has been shown to be upregulated in patients who are EPO-resistant undergoing dialysis.[71] Therapy targeting HCP is attractive, though clinical studies are far away. Similarly, adenovirus-mediated EPO gene therapy which could deliver a stable dose of EPO rather than episodic exogenous EPO treatment is another novel treatment modality.[72] However, no human experiments have been conducted.

Other avenues to increase half-life of exogenous EPO are being explored. For instance, use of synthetic EPO and use of fusion protein, fusing carboxyl-terminal peptide to human chorionic gonadotropin (βHCG) to EPO coding sequence, substantially increased half-life.[73] Human studies are far away in the future.

Different delivery methods are under active investigation, such as a transdermal patch reservoir and oral formulation. Mucoadhesive tablets with absorption augmenter Labrasol (Gattefosse Corp, Saint-Priest, France) have been studied in dogs with improvement in reticulocyte count after a single administration.[74] Pulmonary aerosol delivery of EPO is also being investigated by combining EPO to the Fc protein.[75]

In summary, there are multiple drugs in the pipeline to treat anemia, mainly focusing on modulating the EPO receptor. Given the disappointing experience with the traditional ESAs, the challenge for these agents would be to have acceptable safety profiles.

CONCLUSIONS AND RECOMMENDATIONS

Our understanding of anemia in patients with CKD has undergone significant expansion. The authors have recently urged a revision of the current NKF/KDOQI guidelines. Given the increased risk for CV events and risk for progression of cancer, routine treatment with ESA in otherwise asymptomatic patients who are anemic with CKD can no longer be advocated. After excluding a source of bleeding, correction of iron deficiency with oral iron or cautious administration of IV iron should be the initial approach. Blood transfusions may not be unreasonable, especially in patients with a history of solid tumors or with preexisting cardiovascular disease. Symptomatic patients who are on a transplant list may be one of the subgroups that may require ESA treatment.[76] Which patient sub-population would benefit from ESA remains to be determined. Treatment for patients already on ESA needs to be individualized and targeting Hgb should be avoided. More studies are needed to elucidate the mechanism of higher mortality in patients exposed to ESA as this may give insight into modulating the EPO receptor without inflicting adverse events in this vulnerable patient population. We also do not know the safety and efficacy of ESA in patients who are anemic with CKD in an acute setting. More information is needed on the long-term safety of various IV iron products. Finally, newer treatments targeting different molecules may help expand our armamentarium to treat anemia of CKD.

REFERENCES

1. Foley RN, Parfrey PS, Harnett JD, et al. The impact of anemia on cardiomyopathy, morbidity, and and mortality in end-stage renal disease. Am J Kidney Dis 1996;28:53.

2. Himmelfarb J. Iron regulation. J Am Soc Nephrol 2007;18:379.

3. Andrews NC. Disorders of iron metabolism. N Engl J Med 1999;341:1986.

4. Zhang D, Meyron-Holtz E, Rouault TA. Renal iron metabolism: transferrin iron delivery and the role of iron regulatory proteins. J Am Soc Nephrol 2007; 18:401.

5. Ganz T. Hepcidin, a key regulator of iron metabolism and mediator of anemia of inflammation. Blood 2003;102:783.

6. Weinstein DA, Roy CN, Fleming MD, et al. Inappropriate expression of hepcidin is associated with iron refractory anemia: implications for the anemia of chronic disease. Blood 2002;100:3776.

7. Andrews NC. Forging a field: the golden age of iron biology. Blood 2008;112:219.

8. Nemeth E, Tuttle MS, Powelson J, et al. Hepcidin regulates cellular iron efflux by binding to ferroportin and inducing its internalization. Science 2004;306:2090.

9. Zaritsky J, Young B, Wang HJ, et al. Hepcidin–a potential novel biomarker for iron status in chronic kidney disease. Clin J Am Soc Nephrol 2009;4:1051.

10. Babitt JL, Huang FW, Wrighting DM, et al. Bone morphogenetic protein signaling by hemojuvelin regulates hepcidin expression. Nat Genet 2006;38:531.

11. Niederkofler V, Salie R, Arber S. Hemojuvelin is essential for dietary iron sensing, and its mutation leads to severe iron overload. J Clin Invest 2005; 115:2180.

12. Ekblom P, Thesleff I, Saxen L, et al. Transferrin as a fetal growth factor: acquisition of responsiveness related to embryonic induction. Proc Natl Acad Sci U S A 1983;80:2651.

13. Galy B, Ferring D, Minana B, et al. Altered body iron distribution and microcytosis in mice deficient in iron regulatory protein 2 (IRP2). Blood 2005;106:2580.

14. Alberghini A, Recalcati S, Tacchini L, et al. Loss of the von Hippel Lindau tumor suppressor disrupts iron homeostasis in renal carcinoma cells. J Biol Chem 2005;280:30120.

15. Detivaud L, Nemeth E, Boudjema K, et al. Hepcidin levels in humans are correlated with hepatic iron stores, hemoglobin levels, and hepatic function. Blood 2005;106:746.

16. Valenti L, Girelli D, Valenti GF, et al. HFE mutations modulate the effect of iron on serum hepcidin-25 in chronic hemodialysis patients. Clin J Am Soc Nephrol 2009;4:1331.

17. Ganz T. Molecular control of iron transport. J Am Soc Nephrol 2007;18:394.

18. Kroot JJ, Kemna EH, Bansal SS, et al. Results of the first international round robin for the quantification of urinary and plasma hepcidin assays: need for standardization. Haematologica 2009;94:1748.

19. KDOQI Clinical Practice Guideline and Clinical Practice Recommendations for anemia in chronic kidney disease: 2007 update of hemoglobin target. Am J Kidney Dis 2007;50:471.

20. Fishbane S, Kowalski EA, Imbriano LJ, et al. The evaluation of iron status in hemodialysis patients. J Am Soc Nephrol 1996;7:2654.

21. Coyne DW, Kapoian T, Suki W, et al. Ferric gluconate is highly efficacious in anemic hemodialysis patients with high serum ferritin and low transferrin saturation: results of the Dialysis Patients' Response to IV Iron with Elevated Ferritin (DRIVE) Study. J Am Soc Nephrol 2007;18:975.

22. Singh AK, Coyne DW, Shapiro W, et al. Predictors of the response to treatment in anemic hemodialysis patients with high serum ferritin and low transferrin saturation. Kidney Int 2007;71:1163.

23. National Kidney Foundation. Using iron agents, in KDOQI Clinical Practice Guidelines and Clinical Practice Recommendations for Anemia in Chronic Kidney Disease. Am J Kidney Dis 2006;47:58.

24. Bailie GR, Clark JA, Lane CE, et al. Hypersensitivity reactions and deaths associated with intravenous iron preparations. Nephrol Dial Transplant 2005; 20:1443.

25. Chertow GM, Mason PD, Vaage-Nilsen O, et al. On the relative safety of parenteral iron formulations. Nephrol Dial Transplant 2004;19:1571.

26. Macdougall IC, Roche A. Administration of intravenous iron sucrose as a 2-minute push to CKD patients: a prospective evaluation of 2,297 injections. Am J Kidney Dis 2005;46:283.

27. Michael B, Coyne DW, Fishbane S, et al. Sodium ferric gluconate complex in hemodialysis patients: adverse reactions compared to placebo and iron dextran. Kidney Int 2002;61:1830.

28. Approval of ferumoxytol by FDA - announcement. Available at: http://www.snl.com/irweblinkx/file.aspx?IID=4166432&FID=8015643. Accessed January 15, 2010.

29. Balakrishnan VS, Rao M, Kausz AT, et al. Physicochemical properties of ferumoxytol, a new intravenous iron preparation. Eur J Clin Invest 2009;39:489.

30. Spinowitz BS, Kausz AT, Baptista J, et al. Ferumoxytol for treating iron deficiency anemia in CKD. J Am Soc Nephrol 2008;19:1599.

31. Singh A, Patel T, Hertel J, et al. Safety of ferumoxytol in patients with anemia and CKD. Am J Kidney Dis 2008;52:907.

32. De Domenico I, Ward DM, Kaplan J. Hepcidin regulation: ironing out the details. J Clin Invest 2007;117:1755.

33. Eschbach JW, Egrie JC, Downing MR, et al. Correction of the anemia of end-stage renal disease with recombinant human erythropoietin. Results of a combined phase I and II clinical trial. N Engl J Med 1987;316:73.

34. Wish JB. The economic realities of erythropoiesis-stimulating agent therapy in kidney disease. Kidney Int Suppl 2006;70:S21.

35. Xia H, Ebben J, Ma JZ, et al. Hematocrit levels and hospitalization risks in hemodialysis patients. J Am Soc Nephrol 1999;10:1309.

36. Ma JZ, Ebben J, Xia H, et al. Hematocrit level and associated mortality in hemodialysis patients. J Am Soc Nephrol 1999;10:610.

37. Besarab A, Bolton WK, Browne JK, et al. The effects of normal as compared with low hematocrit values in patients with cardiac disease who are receiving hemodialysis and epoetin. N Engl J Med 1998;339:584.

38. Singh AK, Szczech L, Tang KL, et al. Correction of anemia with epoetin alfa in chronic kidney disease. N Engl J Med 2006;355:2085.

39. Drueke TB, Locatelli F, Clyne N, et al. Normalization of hemoglobin level in patients with chronic kidney disease and anemia. N Engl J Med 2006;355:2071.

40. Foley RN. Target hemoglobin trials in chronic kidney disease: design and interpretation issues. Pediatr Nephrol 2009;24:2279.

41. Phrommintikul A, Haas SJ, Elsik M, et al. Mortality and target haemoglobin concentrations in anaemic patients with chronic kidney disease treated with erythropoietin: a meta-analysis. Lancet 2007;369: 381.

42. Pfeffer MA, Burdmann EA, Chen CY, et al. A trial of darbepoietin alfa in type 2 diabetes and chronic kidney disease. N Engl J Med 2009;361:2019.

43. Fishbane S, Besarab A. Mechanism of increased mortality risk with erythropoietin treatment to higher hemoglobin targets. Clin J Am Soc Nephrol 2007; 2:1274.

44. Szczech LA, Barnhart HX, Inrig JK, et al. Secondary analysis of the CHOIR trial epoetin-alpha dose and achieved hemoglobin outcomes. Kidney Int 2008; 74:791.

45. Keithi-Reddy SR, Addabbo F, Patel TV, et al. Association of anemia and erythropoiesis stimulating agents with inflammatory biomarkers in chronic kidney disease. Kidney Int 2008;74:782.

46. Keithi-Reddy S, Hoppensteadt D, Patel T, et al. Soluble p-selectin, platelet microparticles and cd40 ligand in chronic kidney disease patients on erythropoiesis stimulating agents [SA-PO2805] [abstract]. Am Soc Nephrology Annual Meeting 2008.

47. Parra G, Freddy R, Rosales B, et al. Administration of human recombinant erythropoietin (hrepo) induces systemic oxidative stress [abstract]. J Am Soc Neph 2008.

48. Klinkmann H, Wieczorek L, Scigalla P. Adverse events of subcutaneous recombinant human erythropoietin therapy: results of a controlled multicenter European study. Artif Organs 1993;17:219.

49. Krapf R, Hulter HN. Arterial hypertension induced by erythropoietin and erythropoiesis-stimulating agents (ESA). Clin J Am Soc Nephrol 2009;4:470.

50. Lee MS, Lee JS, Lee JY. Prevention of erythropoietin-associated hypertension. Hypertension 2007; 50:439.

51. Steinbrook R. Erythropoietin, the FDA, and oncology. N Engl J Med 2007;356:2448.

52. Watanabe D, Suzuma K, Matsui S, et al. Erythropoietin as a retinal angiogenic factor in proliferative diabetic retinopathy. N Engl J Med 2005;353:782.

53. Khuri FR. Weighing the hazards of erythropoiesis stimulation in patients with cancer. N Engl J Med 2007;356:2445.

54. Stitt A, McVicar C, Colhoun L, et al. Differential modulation of angiogenesis and pro-inflammatory processes by erythropoiesis-stimulating agents in ischemic retinopathy [abstract]. Am Soc Nephrology Annual Meeting 2008.

55. Agarwal R. Iron, oxidative stress, and clinical outcomes. Pediatr Nephrol 2008;23:1195.

56. Agarwal R, Rizkala AR, Kaskas MO, et al. Iron sucrose causes greater proteinuria than ferric gluconate in non-dialysis chronic kidney disease. Kidney Int 2007;72:638.

57. Zager RA, Johnson AC, Hanson SY. Parenteral iron nephrotoxicity: potential mechanisms and consequences. Kidney Int 2004;66:144.

58. Shah SV, Baliga R, Rajapurkar M, et al. Oxidants in chronic kidney disease. J Am Soc Nephrol 2007; 18:16.

59. Szczech LA, Barnhart HX, Sapp S, et al. A secondary analysis of the CHOIR trial shows that comorbid conditions differentially affect outcomes during anemia treatment. Kidney Int 2010;77:239.

60. Hertel J, Locay H, Scarlata D, et al. Darbepoietin alfa administered every other week maintains hemoglobin levels over 52 weeks in patients with chronic kidney disease converting from once-weekly recombinant human erythropoietin: results from simplify the treatment of anemia with Aranesp (STAAR). Am J Nephrol 2006;26:149.

61. Patel T, Singh A. Treatment of anemia associated with chronic kidney disease with methoxy polyethylene glycol-epoetin beta. Available at: http://www.la-press.com/article.php?article_id=1694; 2009. Accessed January 15, 2010.

62. Stead RB, Lambert J, Wessels D, et al. Evaluation of the safety and pharmacodynamics of Hematide, a novel erythropoietic agent, in a phase 1, double-blind, placebo-controlled, dose-escalation study in healthy volunteers. Blood 2006;108:1830.

63. Zeig S, Geronemus R, Pergola P, et al. Hematide maintains hemoglobin levels in dialysis patients irrespective of gender, age, race, or diabetes as cause of chronic kidney disease [TH-PO726] [abstract]. Am Soc Nephrology Annual Meeting 2008.

64. Locatelli F, Del Vecchio L. Optimizing the management of renal anemia: challenges and new opportunities. Kidney Int Suppl 2008;111:S33.

65. Woodburn KW, Fan Q, Winslow S, et al. Hematide is immunologically distinct from erythropoietin and corrects anemia induced by anti-erythropoietin antibodies in a rat pure red cell aplasia model. Exp Hematol 2007;35:1201.

66. Macdougall IC. Hematide, a novel peptide-based erythropoiesis-stimulating agent for the treatment of anemia. Curr Opin Investig Drugs 2008;9:1034.

67. Nakano Y, Imagawa S, Matsumoto K, et al. Oral administration of K-11706 inhibits GATA binding activity, enhances hypoxia-inducible factor 1 binding activity, and restores indicators in an in vivo mouse model of anemia of chronic disease. Blood 2004;104:4300.

68. Tanaka T, Nangaku M. Drug discovery for overcoming chronic kidney disease (CKD): prolyl-hydroxylase inhibitors to activate hypoxia-inducible factor (HIF) as a novel therapeutic approach in CKD. J Pharmacol Sci 2009;109:24.

69. Guo G, Winmill R, Arend M, et al. Correction of Anemia without Exacerbation of Hypertension in a Rat Model of Chronic Kidney Disease: Comparison of FG-2216 to Recombinant Erythropoietin [SA-PO2422] [abstract]. Am Soc Nephrology Annual Meeting 2008.

70. Available at: http://www.akebia.com/AKB6548_Phase_1a_Completion.pdf. Accessed January 18, 2010.

71. Akagi S, Ichikawa H, Okada T, et al. The critical role of SRC homology domain 2-containing tyrosine phosphatase-1 in recombinant human erythropoietin hyporesponsive anemia in chronic hemodialysis patients. J Am Soc Nephrol 2004;15:3215.

72. Lippin Y, Dranitzki-Elhalel M, Brill-Almon E, et al. Human erythropoietin gene therapy for patients with chronic renal failure. Blood 2005;106:2280.

73. Lee DE, Son W, Ha BJ, et al. The prolonged half-lives of new erythropoietin derivatives via peptide addition. Biochem Biophys Res Commun 2006;339:380.

74. Venkatesan N, Yoshimitsu J, Ohashi Y, et al. Pharmacokinetic and pharmacodynamic studies following oral administration of erythropoietin mucoadhesive tablets to beagle dogs. Int J Pharm 2006;310:46.

75. Bitonti AJ, Dumont JA. Pulmonary administration of therapeutic proteins using an immunoglobulin transport pathway. Adv Drug Deliv Rev 2006;58:1106.

76. Singh AK. Does TREAT give the boot to ESAs in the treatment of CKD anemia? J Am Soc Nephrol 2010; 21:2.

Outcomes Associated with Anemia in Patients with Heart Failure

Adam C. Salisbury, MD, Mikhail Kosiborod, MD*

KEYWORDS

- Heart failure • Anemia • Mortality • Health status
- Outcomes • Treatment • Review

Chronic heart failure (HF) affects 5.7 million people in the United States alone and is a major cause of death, hospital admission, poor physical function, and impaired quality of life.[1,2] In addition to the direct effect of HF on prognosis, medical comorbidities are extremely common in this patient population, particularly among the elderly. The influence of these noncardiovascular conditions on outcomes in patients with HF is receiving increasing attention from researchers and clinicians.[3,4] Of particular interest is anemia, which is common in patients with HF and may represent a modifiable risk factor for adverse outcomes. Increasing awareness of the relationship between anemia and outcomes in these patients has been driven by rapidly growing literature over recent years. The data from these studies show that anemia is associated with a broad range of outcomes, including poorer survival, more frequent hospitalization, and worse health status in patients with HF.[5–10] This article summarizes the current data with regard to the prevalence of anemia in patients with HF and the association between anemia and clinical outcomes.

PREVALENCE OF ANEMIA IN PATIENTS WITH HF

Across diverse populations of patients with HF and various care settings, estimates of the prevalence of anemia range from as low as 4% to as high as 61% and have been described in detail in several earlier reviews (**Table 1**).[11–16] Although most investigations have focused on patients who have impaired systolic function, prevalence is similar in patients with HF with preserved systolic function.[8,17] Most estimates place the prevalence of anemia at more than 20% in ambulatory and hospitalized populations. Pooling 34 studies that evaluated the relationship between anemia and mortality in a meta-analysis of anemia in HF, Groenveld and colleagues[5] reported the overall prevalence of 37.2%.

Several factors explain the variation in prevalence across these studies. The definition of anemia has varied widely across studies, although the World Health Organization (WHO) definition (hemoglobin [Hgb] level<13 g/dL in men, <12 g/dL in women) has been used most commonly.[18] More restrictive definitions often result in significantly lower estimates. Study type also strongly influences prevalence because the prevalence of anemia in more selected clinical trial cohorts[6,7,19] is typically lower than estimates reported by observational registries[20] and analyses of administrative data.[16] For example, using the same WHO definition, the prevalence of anemia obtained from randomized trial cohorts such as Valsartan Heart Failure Trial (Val-HeFT) (23%)[7] and the Carvedilol or Metoprolol European Trial (COMET) (16%)[6] is lower than that obtained from unselected registries such as Study of Anemia in a Heart Failure Population (STAMINA-HFP)[20] (34%) and administrative studies such as the Anemia in

Saint Luke's Mid-America Heart Institute Cardiovascular Outcomes Research (MAHI HI-5), 4401 Wornall Road, Kansas City, MO 64111, USA
* Corresponding author.
E-mail address: mkosiborod@cc-pc.com

Heart Failure Clin 6 (2010) 359–372
doi:10.1016/j.hfc.2010.03.005
1551-7136/10/$ – see front matter © 2010 Elsevier Inc. All rights reserved.

Table 1
The prevalence of anemia and the relationship between anemia and mortality (selected sample of larger studies)

Study	Sample Size	Follow-up Duration	Study Type	Patient Population	Anemia Definition	Prevalence	Adjusted Mortality Risk[a]
Al-Ahmad et al,[11] 2001	6635	33 mo	Clinical trial cohort	EF<35%, symptomatic or asymptomatic	Hct<35% or Hct<39%	4% (Hct<35%) and 22% (Hct<39%)	HR, 1.03 (95% CI, 1.02–1.04) per 1% lower Hct
Horwich, et al,[9] 2002	1061	12 mo	Retrospective cohort	Single-center HF management program	Hgb<13.0 g/dL in men, Hgb<12 g/dL in women	30%	RR, 1.13 (95% CI, 1.05–1.22) per 1 g/dL lower Hgb
McClellan et al,[30] 2002	633	12 mo	Retrospective cohort	Medicare beneficiaries admitted with HF	Hct<36%	47%	HR, 1.07 (95% CI, 0.59–1.9)
Ezekowitz et al,[23] 2003	12,065	19 mo	Administrative data analysis	Patients discharged with new-onset HF	Discharge ICD-9 codes	17%	HR, 1.34 (95% CI, 1.24–1.46)
Felker et al,[44] 2003	906	2 mo	Clinical trial cohort	CHF exacerbation, systolic dysfunction	Hgb<13.0 g/dL in men, Hgb <12 g/dL in women	49%	Composite death/rehospitalization: OR, 0.89 (95% CI, 0.82–0.91) per 1 g/dL higher Hgb
Kalra et al,[31] 2003	531	36 mo	Prospective cohort	New-onset HF referred to HF clinic	Hgb<13.0 g/dL	36%	HR, 0.98 (95% CI, 0.92–1.04) per 1 g/dL higher Hgb
Kosiborod et al,[25] 2003	2281	12 mo	Retrospective cohort	Medicare beneficiaries admitted with HF	Hct<37%	48%	HR, 1.02 (95% CI, 1.01–1.04) per 1% lower Hct

Study	N	Follow-up	Study type	Patient population	Anemia definition	Prevalence	Outcome
Mozaffarian et al,[45] 2003	1130	15 mo	Clinical trial cohort	EF≤30%, NYHA class III or IV HF	Hct<37.6%	20%	HR, 1.52 (95% CI, 1.11–2.10)
Anand et al,[26] 2004	912	13 mo	Clinical trial cohort	EF≤30%, NYHA II–IV HF symptoms	Hgb<12 g/dL	12%	HR, 0.84 (P = .0009) per 1 g/dL Hgb increase[b]
Sharma et al,[24] 2004	3044	18 mo	Clinical trial cohort	EF≤40%, age>60 y	Hgb<12 g/dL	17%	RR, 1.24 (95% CI, 1.01–1.52)
Ezekowitz et al,[46] 2005	791	60 mo	Prospective cohort	Ambulatory patients referred to a specialty HF clinic	Hgb<13.0 g/dL in men, Hgb <12 g/dL in women	39%	HR, 1.76, (95% CI, 1.15–2.70) in men; HR, 1.15 (95% CI, 0.65–2.05) in women
Ishani et al,[19] 2005	6436	12 mo	Clinical trial cohort	EF<35%, asymptomatic or symptomatic	Hct<39% in men, Hct <36 in women	18% (incident cases of anemia developed in 10% during 1 y)	Prevalent anemia: HR, 1.44 (95% CI, 1.27–1.64) (Incident anemia: HR, 2.08 [95% CI, 1.82–2.38])
Kosiborod et al,[16] 2005	50,405	12 mo	Retrospective cohort	Medicare beneficiaries hospitalized with HF	Hct<40% for men, Hct<37% for women	61% of men, 52% of women	Hct>36%–40%: RR, 1.04 (95% CI, 0.98–1.10); Hct>32%–36%: RR, 1.09 (95% CI, 1.03–1.16); Hct>28%–32%: RR, 1.13 (95% CI, 1.05–1.20); Hct>24%–28%: RR, 0.99 (95% CI, 0.89–1.09); Hct<24%: RR, 1.02 (95% CI, 0.86–1.19)

(continued on next page)

Table 1
(continued)

Study	Sample Size	Follow-up Duration	Study Type	Patient Population	Anemia Definition	Prevalence	Adjusted Mortality Risk[a]
Maggioni et al,[47] 2005	2411 (IN-CHF); 5010 (Val-HeFT)	12 mo (IN-CHF); 23 mo (Val-HeFT)	Retrospective cohort (IN-CHF); Clinical trial cohort (Val-HeFT)	Ambulatory patients at cardiology centers (IN-CHF); Stable NYHA II–IV symptoms, EF ≤40% (Val-HeFT)	Hgb<12 g/dL in men, Hgb<11 g/dL in women	16% (IN-CHF) 10% (Val-HeFT)	HR, 1.54 (95% CI, 1.20–1.97) (IN-CHF) HR, 1.26 (95% CI, 1.04–1.52) in Val-HeFT
Go et al,[21] 2006	59,772	25 mo	Administrative, Kaiser chronic HF cohort	Ambulatory or hospitalized patients with diagnosis of HF	Hgb<13.0 g/dL in men, Hgb<12 g/dL in women	43%	Compared with reference category Hgb, 13.0–13.9 g/dL: Hgb, 12.0–12.9 g/dL: HR, 1.16 (95% CI, 1.11–1.21) Hgb, 11.0–11.9 g/dL: HR, 1.50 (95% CI, 1.44–1.57) Hgb, 10.0–10.9 g/dL: HR, 1.89 (95% CI, 1.80–1.98) Hgb, 9.0–9.9 g/dL: HR, 2.31 (95% CI, 2.18–2.45) Hgb<9.0 g/dL: HR, 3.48 (95% CI, 3.25–3.73)
Komajda et al,[6] 2006	2996	58 mo	Clinical trial cohort	NYHA II–IV symptoms, EF<35, prior cardiac admission	Hgb<13.0 g/dL in men, Hgb<12 g/dL in women	16%	Compared with reference category Hgb, 13.0–14.0 g/dL: Hgb<11.5 g/dL: RR, 1.56 (95% CI, 1.15–2.12) Hgb, 11.5–13.0 g/dL: RR, 1.41 (95% CI, 1.16–1.70)

Source	No. of Patients	Study Design	Definition of HF/Population	Follow-up	Definition of Anemia	Prevalence of Anemia	Outcome
Maraldi et al,[32] 2006	567	Prospective cohort	Diagnosis of HF, age>65 y, admitted to internal medicine or geriatric wards	10 mo	Hgb<13.0 g/dL in men, Hgb<12 g/dL in women	45%	HR, 1.15 (95% CI, 0.69–1.91)
O'Meara et al,[8] 2006	2653	Clinical trial cohort	NYHA class II–IV symptoms, systolic or diastolic dysfunction (CHARM-Preserved)	Outcomes reported per 1000 patient y of follow-up	Hgb<13.0 g/dL in men, Hgb<12 g/dL in women	26%	RR, 1.94 (P<.001)[b,c]
Valeur et al,[48] 2006	1731	Clinical trial cohort	Post-MI patients with EF≤35%	10 y	Hgb<13.0 g/dL in men, Hgb<12 g/dL in women	25%	HR, 1.06 (95% CI, 0.93–1.21) in all patients with anemia vs no anemia HR, 1.16 (95% CI, 1.01–1.34) in patients who developed HF
Varadarajan et al,[49] 2006	2246	Retrospective, single-center cohort	Discharge ICD-9 codes for CHF with an echocardiogram during admission or within 1 mo prior	60 mo	Hgb<12 g/dL	45%	Preserved systolic function: HR, 1.23 (1.02–1.49) per 1 g/dL lower Hgb Depressed ejection fraction: HR, 1.24 (95% CI, 1.02–1.51)
Dunlay et al,[50] 2008	1063 (retrospective) 677 (prospective)	Retrospective and prospective cohort	Retrospective: incident HF Prospective: active HF confirmed by Framingham criteria	60 mo (retrospective) 20 mo (prospective)	Hgb<13.0 g/dL in men, Hgb <12 g/dL in women	40% (retrospective) 53% (prospective)	Prospective: reference category Hgb, 14.0–15.9 g/dL Hgb, 12–13.9 g/dL: HR, 1.41 (95% CI, 0.89–2.31) Hgb, 10–11.9 g/dL: HR, 1.99 (95% CI, 1.27–3.25) Hgb<10 g/dL: HR, 2.37 (95% CI, 1.39–4.11)
Kawashiro et al,[51] 2008	3578	Retrospective cohort	Patients admitted with HF confirmed by Framingham criteria	34 mo	Hgb<14.0 g/dL in men; Hgb<12.0 g/dL in women	44%	HR, 1.46 (95% CI, 1.18–1.80)

(continued on next page)

Table 1
(continued)

Study	Sample Size	Follow-up Duration	Study Type	Patient Population	Anemia Definition	Prevalence	Adjusted Mortality Risk[a]
Tang et al,[33] 2008	6159	47 mo	Retrospective cohort	Ambulatory, consecutive patients with HF at a single center	Hgb<12.0 g/dL in men; Hgb<11.0 g/dL in women	17%	RR, 0.85 (95% CI, 0.77–0.94) per 1 g/dL higher Hgb
Young et al,[36] 2008	48,612 (mortality based on follow-up data, n = 5791)	2–3 mo	Prospective multicenter cohort	Hospitalized with new or worsening HF, preserved or depressed EF	Hgb<10.7 g/dL Hgb<12.1 g/dL	25% (Hgb <10.7 g/dL) 51% (Hgb <12.1 g/dL)	OR, 1.08 (95% CI, 1.08–1.13) per 1 g/dL lower Hgb up to 13 g/dL
Anker et al,[52] 2009	5010	12 mo	Clinical trial cohort	AMI complicated by signs/symptoms of HF	Hgb<13.0 g/dL in men, Hgb<12 g/dL in women	27% (incidence during 1 y, 10%)	HR, 0.88 (95% CI, 0.83–0.93) per 1 SD higher Hgb
Hamaguchi et al,[53] 2009	1960	26 mo	Prospective cohort	Patients hospitalized with worsening HF	Hgb<13.0 g/dL in men, Hgb<12 g/dL in women	57%	Compared with the reference category of Hgb>13.7 g/dL Hgb<10.1 g/dL: HR, 1.96 (95% CI, 1.30–2.96) Hgb 10.1–11.9: HR, 1.61 (95% CI, 1.07–2.42)
Peterson et al,[34] 2010	2478	16 mo	Prospective cohort	Patients discharged with diagnosis of HF	Hgb<13.0 g/dL in men, Hgb<12 g/dL in women	45%	Prevalent anemia: HR, 1.11 (95% CI, 0.97–1.28) Persistent anemia: HR, 1.65 (95% CI, 1.27–2.14) Decline in Hgb vs persistent nonanemic: HR, 1.54 (95% CI, 1.16–2.05)

Selected large (n>500) studies of anemia and mortality in patients with HF.

Abbreviations: AMI, acute myocardial infarction; CHARM, Candesartan in Heart Failure: Assessment of Reduction in Mortality and Morbidity; CHF, congestive heart failure; CI, confidence interval; EF, ejection fraction; Hct, hematocrit; Hgb, hemoglobin; HR, hazard ratio; ICD, International Classification of Diseases; IN-CHF, Italian Network on Congestive Heart Failure registry; NYHA, New York Heart Association; OR, odds ratio; RR, risk ratio; Val-HeFT, Valsartan Heart Failure Trial.

[a] Comparisons listed are between anemia versus no anemia unless otherwise specified.
[b] Adjusted data not reported.
[c] Calculated from data in the manuscript (132.9 deaths/1000 person years in anemic patients vs 68.6 deaths/1000 person years in nonanemic patients).

Chronic Heart Failure: Outcomes and Resource Utilization (ANCHOR) cohort (43%).[21] Characteristics such as the age and gender of patients studied, race, locus of enrollment (inpatients vs ambulatory), New York Heart Association (NYHA) class, and burden of comorbid diseases, such as renal failure, in the population studied also have a profound influence on prevalence estimates.[12,14,15] In particular, age, gender, and race are so strongly related to anemia that Beutler and Waalen[22] have proposed new diagnostic criteria for anemia accounting for these factors for all patient populations with anemia. Using these criteria, a white man aged between 20 and 59 years would be considered anemic at an Hgb level of less than a threshold value of 13.7 g/dL, whereas a black woman of the same age would not be considered anemic unless her Hgb level were less than 11.5 g/dL.

The relationships between many of these demographic and clinical patient characteristics and prevalence of anemia are robust and have been demonstrated to persist after multivariable adjustment. For example, Ezekowitz and colleagues[23] reported that greater age, female sex, chronic kidney disease, and hypertension were independent correlates of anemia in a population-based cohort of patients with new-onset HF.

THE ASSOCIATION BETWEEN ANEMIA AND MORTALITY

Over the last decade, numerous well-conducted studies have demonstrated strong relationships between anemia and survival in populations with HF, ranging from clinical trial cohorts, observational registries, and administrative datasets to community-based studies. Regardless of the definition, anemia consistently portends a poor prognosis. Adjusted associations between anemia and mortality from a selected sample of earlier studies are shown in **Table 1**, and several points merit further discussion. When analyzed as a dichotomous variable, adjusted estimates for the association between anemia and mortality vary from nonsignificant to robust, with most point estimates indicating a 24% to 94% increase in the risk for death for patients with anemia.[8,24] When the association of each 1-g/dL change in Hgb with mortality is reported, point estimates range from a 2% increase in 1-year mortality with a 1 g/dL Hgb decline[25] to a 16% improved survival with a 1 g/dL improvement in Hgb.[26] When studies were grouped based on categories of anemia severity, they showed graded, incremental increases in adjusted mortality risk with declining Hgb, from a hazard ratio (HR)of 1.16 (95%

confidence interval [CI], 1.11–1.21) for mild anemia (Hgb level of 12.0–12.9 g/dL) to an HR of 3.48 (95% CI, 3.25–3.73) for severe anemia (Hgb level<9 g/dL).[21]

Many studies that have examined the association between anemia and mortality were analyzed in a comprehensive meta-analysis performed by Groenveld and colleagues.[5] Using random effects meta-analysis, the investigators examined the relationship between anemia and mortality among 34 studies with 153,180 patients. The duration of follow-up in the included studies ranged from at least 6 months to as long as 5 years, and most of these investigations used the WHO definition of anemia (Hgb level<13.0 g/dL in men, <12.0 g/dL in women). The investigators used the anemia definitions of the original studies and examined the association between anemia as a dichotomous variable and mortality. The unadjusted risk for mortality (odds ratio [OR], 1.96; 95% CI, 1.78–2.14, $P<.001$) was significantly higher for patients with anemia than for those without anemia (**Fig. 1**). Exclusion of the 2 largest studies (Go and colleagues,[21] N = 59,772 and Kosiborod and colleagues,[16] N = 50,405) did not alter the mortality risk estimate, indicating that the point estimate of mortality risk was not unduly influenced by these large administrative cohorts. Mortality risk was similar in patients with systolic HF (OR, 1.96; 95% CI, 1.70–2.25, $P<.001$) and patients with diastolic HF (OR, 2.09; 95% CI, 1.53–2.86, $P<.001$). There was no evidence of publication bias, and although there was significant heterogeneity between included studies, this was largely attributable to the definition of anemia used. Adjusted mortality risks were available for 127,437 (83.1% of total) patients, and all but one study adjusted for important covariates such as age and renal function. In these analyses, anemia was independently associated with a 46% increase in the risk for death (HR, 1.46; 95% CI, 1.26–1.69, $P<.001$). Finally, the investigators reported results of metaregression analyses identifying an inverse relationship between creatinine and the influence of anemia on mortality. This result reflects that at higher creatinine levels, renal disease accounts for a greater proportion of the mortality risk than anemia (which is likely a marker for advanced renal disease in these patients).

Although these observational data are important, they do not provide a definitive answer to a key question: whether anemia is directly harmful in patients with HF or whether it is simply a marker of greater disease severity and comorbidity burden. Pathophysiologic data suggest several potential mechanisms by which anemia could mediate poor outcomes,[15,27] including its

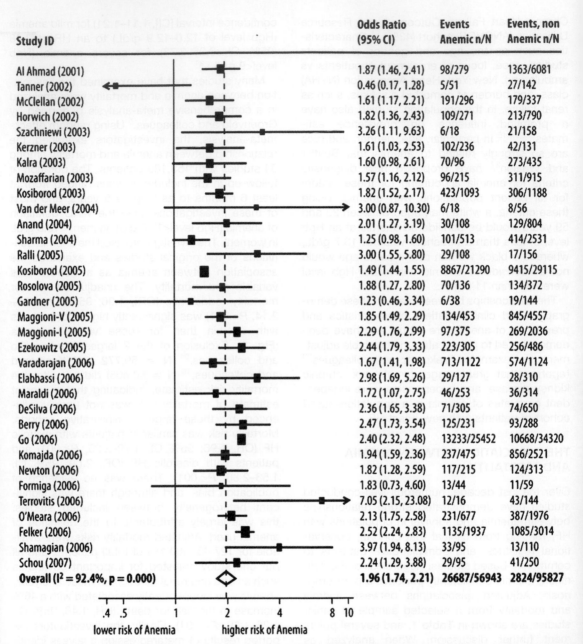

Study ID	Odds Ratio (95% CI)	Events Anemic n/N	Events, non Anemic n/N
Al Ahmad (2001)	1.87 (1.46, 2.41)	98/279	1363/6081
Tanner (2002)	0.46 (0.17, 1.28)	5/51	27/142
McClellan (2002)	1.61 (1.17, 2.21)	191/296	179/337
Horwich (2002)	1.82 (1.36, 2.43)	109/271	213/790
Szachniewi (2003)	3.26 (1.11, 9.63)	6/18	21/158
Kerzner (2003)	1.61 (1.03, 2.53)	102/236	42/131
Kalra (2003)	1.60 (0.98, 2.61)	70/96	273/435
Mozaffarian (2003)	1.57 (1.16, 2.12)	96/215	311/915
Kosiborod (2003)	1.82 (1.52, 2.17)	423/1093	306/1188
Van der Meer (2004)	3.00 (0.87, 10.30)	6/18	8/56
Anand (2004)	2.01 (1.27, 3.19)	30/108	129/804
Sharma (2004)	1.25 (0.98, 1.60)	101/513	414/2531
Ralli (2005)	3.00 (1.55, 5.80)	29/108	17/156
Kosiborod (2005)	1.49 (1.44, 1.55)	8867/21290	9415/29115
Rosolova (2005)	1.88 (1.27, 2.80)	70/136	134/372
Gardner (2005)	1.23 (0.46, 3.34)	6/38	19/144
Maggioni-V (2005)	1.85 (1.49, 2.29)	134/453	845/4557
Maggioni-I (2005)	2.29 (1.76, 2.99)	97/375	269/2036
Ezekowitz (2005)	2.44 (1.79, 3.33)	223/305	256/486
Varadarajan (2006)	1.67 (1.41, 1.98)	713/1122	574/1124
Elabbassi (2006)	2.98 (1.69, 5.26)	29/127	28/310
Maraldi (2006)	1.72 (1.07, 2.75)	46/253	36/314
DeSilva (2006)	2.36 (1.65, 3.38)	71/305	74/650
Berry (2006)	2.47 (1.73, 3.54)	125/231	93/288
Go (2006)	2.40 (2.32, 2.48)	13233/25452	10668/34320
Komajda (2006)	1.94 (1.59, 2.36)	237/475	856/2521
Newton (2006)	1.82 (1.28, 2.59)	117/215	124/313
Formiga (2006)	1.83 (0.73, 4.60)	13/44	11/59
Terrovitis (2006)	7.05 (2.15, 23.08)	12/16	43/144
O'Meara (2006)	2.13 (1.75, 2.58)	231/677	387/1976
Felker (2006)	2.52 (2.24, 2.83)	1135/1937	1085/3014
Shamagian (2006)	3.97 (1.94, 8.13)	33/95	13/110
Schou (2007)	2.24 (1.29, 3.88)	29/95	41/250
Overall (I^2 = 92.4%, p = 0.000)	1.96 (1.74, 2.21)	26687/56943	2824/95827

.4 .5   1   2   4   8 10

lower risk of Anemia   higher risk of Anemia

Fig. 1. All-cause mortality in patients with HF with and without anemia. (*From* Groenveld HF, Januzzi JL, Damman K, et al. Anemia and mortality in patients with HF: a systematic review and meta-analysis. J Am Coll Cardiol 2008;52(10):818–27, copyright 2008, Elsevier; with permission.)

hemodynamic and neurohormonal effects.[28,29] However, in several studies, higher mortality was observed even with modest declines in Hgb levels that were higher than the levels thought to mediate direct pathophysiologic decompensation, casting some doubt on whether the observed relationship between anemia and mortality is mediated through these mechanisms. Furthermore, patients with anemia often have a substantially greater comorbidity burden than those without anemia; thus,

the association between a lower Hgb level and worse survival could potentially be because of residual (unmeasured) confounding. Supporting this notion, several investigators have demonstrated that the association between anemia and mortality is significantly attenuated when the statistical models adjust for extensive range and severity of noncardiac comorbidities. In fact, some have found that this relationship is no longer significant after full adjustment for these important covariates.[16,30–32] In the largest of these investigations, a cohort of Medicare recipients hospitalized with HF was followed up for 1 year to compare mortality and rehospitalization rates between anemic and nonanemic patients. In unadjusted analyses, a graded increase in the risk for death was observed with progressively lower hematocrit (Hct). However, after extensive adjustment for demographic, noncardiac, and cardiovascular comorbidities; HF severity; laboratory values; vital signs; and admission medications, severe anemia was no longer independently associated with worse survival.[16] Although these findings suggest that anemia may be predominantly a marker for "sicker patients," this issue continues to be a subject of intense debate and will not be completely resolved until randomized clinical trials establish whether correction of anemia has any effect on patient outcomes. Regardless, anemia remains important in evaluation of an individual patient's risk given the ease and availability of Hgb assessments in clinical practice.

CHANGE IN HEMOGLOBIN LEVELS OVER TIME AND MORTALITY

Because Hgb levels and anemia status vary over time, it is important to understand the relationship between dynamic changes in Hgb level and mortality. Although most earlier investigations evaluated anemia status at a single point in time, several studies offer insights into the prognostic value of temporal changes in Hgb levels. Post hoc analyses from the Val-HeFT and COMET trials reported a relationship between change in Hgb level and survival. Anand and colleagues[7] analyzed the data from the Val-HeFT clinical trial by dividing patients into quartiles of Hgb level change during 12 months. Patients in the quartile with the greatest decline in Hgb level (mean reduction of 1.64 g/dL) had a 60% greater adjusted risk for death in comparison with patients with the smallest change ($P = .004$). An increase in Hgb level of 1 g/dL in this study was associated with a reduced adjusted mortality risk in patients with and without anemia at baseline (anemic patients: HR, 0.78; 95% CI, 0.65–0.93; nonanemic patients: HR, 0.79; 95% CI, 0.71–0.89). Similarly, in an analysis of the COMET trial cohort, large declines in Hgb level of 2 to 3 g/dl and greater than 3 g/dl were independently associated with greater mortality (risk ratio [RR], 1.47; 95% CI, 1.09–1.97 and RR, 3.37; 95% CI, 2.46–4.61, respectively) compared with patients whose Hgb level did not change or increased by 1 g/dL or less.[6] More modest decreases or increases in Hgb levels were not significantly associated with mortality in comparison with the reference group.

Additional insights from a retrospective analysis of outpatients with HF receiving care at the Cleveland Clinic suggest that prognosis is strongly related to resolution or persistence of anemia. Tang and colleagues[33] compared baseline and 6-month Hgb levels and assessed effect of persistence, resolution, or new development of anemia on long-term outcomes during a mean follow-up of 5 years. Patients with persistent anemia had a worse survival rate than those whose anemia resolved, those with new-onset anemia, or those without anemia at baseline (**Fig. 2**). Moreover, Petersen and colleagues[34] found that longitudinal changes in the level of Hgb were prognostically more important than a baseline assessment. The trajectory analyses demonstrated that temporal changes in Hgb levels were common; in fact, more than one-third of the cohort had variable patterns of anemia. Mortality rate was greater in patients with persistently low Hgb level (HR, 1.65; 95% CI, 1.27–2.14) and with further decline (HR, 1.54; 95% CI, 1.16–2.05) compared with those who had no anemia at baseline or during follow-up. Despite these data, it remains unclear whether improving the level of Hgb directly improves survival or whether this clinical pattern simply identifies patients who are less ill or have a transient cause of anemia (eg, bleeding) leading to different prognosis from the "sicker" patients with persistent or progressive anemia.

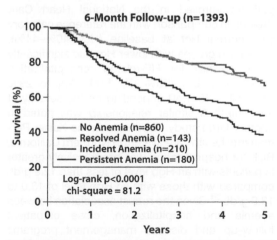

Fig. 2. All-cause mortality among outpatients with HF with no anemia, persistent anemia, resolved anemia, and incident anemia during 6 months of follow-up. (*From* Tang WHW, Tong W, Jain A, et al. Evaluation and long-term prognosis of new-onset, transient, and persistent anemia in patients with chronic heart failure. J Am Coll Cardiol 2008;51(5):569–76, copyright 2008, Elsevier; with permission.)

ASSOCIATION OF ANEMIA WITH HOSPITALIZATION

Hospital admission is an important outcome that has received increasing focus given extremely high rates of repeat hospitalizations in the patient population with HF (24.4% median 30-day readmission rate across hospitals caring for Medicare beneficiaries with HF).[35] Admissions for HF have the potential to dramatically increase cost to the health care system and negatively affect patients' quality of life and are more common in patients with anemia. Analyses of several randomized trial cohorts have shown a relationship between anemia and increased risk for repeat hospitalization for HF.[6–8] Specifically, Komajda and colleagues[6] reported that anemia was independently associated with increased all-cause hospitalization (severe anemia: HR, 1.72 [95% CI, 1.34–2.21]; moderate anemia: HR, 1.22 [95% CI, 1.05–1.42]) and hospitalization for worsening HF (HR, 1.70 [95% CI, 1.22–2.36]; moderate anemia: HR, 1.47 [95% CI, 1.21–1.80]) in the COMET study. Data from patients in the more generalizable Organized Program to Initiate Lifesaving Treatment in Patients with Heart Failure (OPTIMIZE-HF) registry also indicate that the risk for hospital readmission increases with a lower baseline Hgb level (60–90 day readmission rate of 33.1% in the lowest Hgb quartile [Hgb<10.7 g/dL] vs 24.2% in the highest quartile [Hgb>13.5 g/dL], P<.001).[36] The independent association between anemia and repeat hospitalization also persisted even after extensive multivariable adjustment in the analysis of 50,405 patients enrolled in the National Heart Care Project. In comparison with the reference category with normal Hct at baseline (Hct, 40%–44%), patients in groups with lower Hct had significantly increased risk for HF-related rehospitalization (range from 9% [95% CI, 1.09–1.22] to 29% [95% CI, 1.18–1.40 depending on the severity of anemia]).[16] A similar relationship was noted in another large study of patients in the Kaiser Permanente health care system in Northern California. Risk for hospitalization was progressively greater in patients with an Hgb level of less than 12.9 g/dL compared with those with an Hgb level of 13.0 to 13.9 g/dL.[21] Given the robust association between anemia and hospitalization, close outpatient follow-up and disease management programs may need to be considered in anemic patients after hospitalization for HF; this approach may help to avert hospital readmission through early recognition and management of worsening clinical status. Moreover, readmission should be an important outcome of interest for future studies on anemia treatment. Specifically, given the clinical and economic impact of recurrent hospitalizations for HF, there is a need to better understand whether correction of anemia may decrease readmission rates.

ANEMIA AND HOSPITAL PERFORMANCE MEASURES

In addition to mortality and readmission data, a report from OPTIMIZE-HF contains interesting data on the relationship between anemia and achievement of hospital performance measures.[36] Patients in the lowest quartile of Hgb level (<10.7 g/dL) were less likely to have documentation of several HF performance measures, including discharge prescription of angiotensin-converting (ACE) inhibitors and β-blockers, receipt of smoking cessation counseling or complete discharge instructions, or assessment of left ventricular ejection fraction during admission (all P<.01). Although these comparisons are not adjusted for important confounders (eg, blood pressure with regard to ACE inhibitor and β-blocker use), they do provide initial insights into the relationship between anemia and an outcome that has received little attention in this patient population. It is unclear whether these findings are a reflection of a much greater burden of comorbidity and HF complications in anemic patients or if anemia is independently associated with poorer provision of care in-hospital. Nevertheless, this "risk-treatment paradox" (wherein sicker patients who may benefit most from life-saving interventions receive less optimal care) may partially explain worse outcomes in anemic patients with HF and warrants further study.

HEALTH STATUS OUTCOMES OF ANEMIC PATIENTS WITH HF

HF has a profound effect on patients' symptoms, function, and quality of life, and health status is increasingly recognized as a critical outcome in evaluation of patients with HF. Health status is important as the primary concern of many patients with HF and has also been shown to be predictive of long-term outcomes, such as mortality and hospitalization.[37,38] Surprisingly, few investigations have focused on the relationship between anemia and health status despite the availability of several validated disease-specific instruments of health status assessment.

The NYHA classification system remains the most frequently used tool for clinical assessment of symptoms of patients with HF and should be sensitive to the potential influence of anemia. A study by Horwich and colleagues[9] evaluated patients enrolled in a HF management program between 1983 and 1999 and found a significant association between anemia and NYHA class. Among patients in the lowest Hgb quartile (<12.3 g/dL), 75% had class IV symptoms compared with 68% in quartile 2 (Hgb level, 12.3–13.6 g/dL), 57% in quartile 3 (Hgb level, 13.7–14.7 g/dL), and 59% in patients with Hgb level of more than 14.8 g/dL (P<.0001). Data from other studies including randomized trials and observational studies also reveal that the proportion of patients with NYHA class III and IV HF is higher in patients with anemia than in patients without anemia.[6–8,20]

Disease-specific measures, such as the Minnesota Living with Heart Failure Questionnaire (MLHFQ) and the Kansas City Cardiomyopathy Questionnaire (KCCQ), are particularly important tools to assess the effect of anemia on HF. Importantly, the KCCQ has been specifically evaluated and found to be valid, reliable, and responsive to clinical change in patients with HF and anemia.[39] In this study, the KCCQ was used to quantify the relationship between changes in Hct and health status in 1382 patients enrolled in the Eplerenone's Neurohormonal Efficacy and Survival Study (EPHESUS) quality-of-life substudy. A significant cross-sectional association between lower Hct and worse baseline health status was noted. The effect of change in Hct on change in health status was assessed by comparing change in Hct and health status between baseline (1-month outpatient assessment) and 3-month follow-up assessments.[40] A nonlinear relationship between health status and Hct was described, whereby patients who were anemic and baseline and who suffered further decline in Hct experienced declining health status. In contrast, modest health status improvements were noted in patients who were severely anemic but had higher Hct at 3 months, and no significant improvement in health status was observed in those with mild-to-moderate anemia at baseline and subsequent recovery of Hct during follow-up. Change in Hct was not associated with change in health status among patients with normal Hct at baseline.

Adams and colleagues[10] evaluated the effect of anemia on health status using the KCCQ and the MLHFQ in the STAMINA-HFP cohort. At baseline, the investigators found a significant, independent relationship between Hgb level and health status as assessed by all domains of the KCCQ and the MLHFQ. They also examined the effect of changes in Hgb level over time on health status. At each follow-up time point, an increase in Hgb level of 1 g/dL or more was associated with a large increase in KCCQ clinical score, whereas less than 1 g/dL increase or decrease in Hgb level

was associated with modest improvements in KCCQ score, and decline in Hgb level of more than 1 g/dL was associated with worsening KCCQ clinical score (**Fig. 3**).

Disability represents an extreme along the spectrum of functional status, and anemia also seems to be strongly related with its development. Maraldi and colleagues[32] studied a cohort of elderly, nondisabled patients admitted with HF; disability

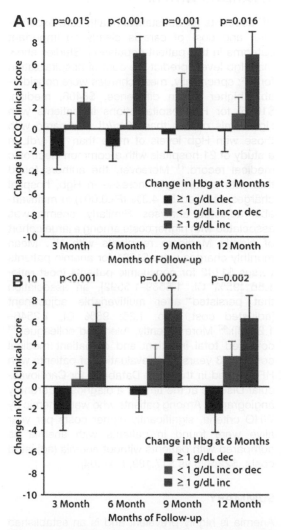

Fig. 3. Relationship between change in Hgb levels and adjusted change in KCCQ clinical score from baseline to follow-up time points. (*A*) Change in hemoglobin levels from baseline to 3 months. (*B*) Change in hemoglobin levels from baseline to 6 months. Results are displayed as mean ± standard error of the mean. inc, increase; dec, decrease. (*From* Adams KF, Pina IL, Ghali JK, et al. Prospective evaluation of the association between hemoglobin concentration and quality of life in patients with heart failure. Am Heart J 2009;158(6):965–71, copyright 2009, Elsevier; with permission.)

was defined as a dependence on others for completion of at least 2 activities of daily living. Anemia was strongly associated with the development of disability at 1 year (adjusted OR, 2.17 [95% CI, 1.12–4.24]); this relationship was particularly pronounced in women (OR, 2.62 [95% CI, 1.06–6.50]).

ANEMIA AND COST OF CARE IN PATIENTS WITH HF

HF accounts for substantial health care expenditure, and cost of care is clearly an important outcome in this patient population. Studies show that Hgb levels predict the cost of hospitalization for HF; specifically, mean charges were considerably higher (mean difference, $8406; median, $1915) for HF hospitalizations in patients with Hgb levels of less than 10 g/dL compared with those with Hgb levels of more than 12 g/dL in a study of 21 hospitals with a common electronic medical record.[41] Moreover, the authors found that with each 1 g/dl increase in Hgb, hospital charges declined by 4.3% ($P<0.001$) in multivariable adjusted analyses. Similarly, anemia was associated with higher costs among a large cohort of elderly Medicare recipients with HF. Mean monthly charges were $1781 for anemic patients versus $1142 for nonanemic patients (cost ratio, 1.56 [95% CI, 1.5589–1.5592], an association that persisted after multivariable adjustment [adjusted cost ratio, 1.25; 95% CI, 1.2546–1.2548]).[42] More recently, Allen and colleagues[43] collected total inpatient and outpatient medical costs for 3 years in an evaluation of patients with HF enrolled in the Duke Databank for Cardiovascular Disease at the time of a diagnostic coronary angiography. Among patients who were anemic by WHO criteria, significantly higher costs per year alive were found in patients with anemia as compared with patients without anemia (adjusted costs, $22,926 vs $17,189, $P = .04$).

SUMMARY

Anemia is highly prevalent and is an established risk factor for poor survival, frequent hospitalization, and impaired health status in patients with HF. Despite these associations, it is unclear whether anemia is directly harmful or is a marker for greater disease severity and comorbidity burden. Clinical studies of anemia correction in this patient population have been limited, and the risk-benefit balance of this therapeutic approach remains to be fully defined. In the interim, careful consideration of the Hgb levels of patients with HF is useful for risk stratification and could help

clinicians identify a particularly high-risk subset of patients that may benefit from close follow-up. Furthermore, careful evaluation of the cause of anemia is warranted in these patients because many suffer from iron deficiency that is easily treatable. Well-designed trials that are appropriately powered to evaluate meaningful clinical outcomes are needed to clarify whether optimization of Hgb levels can safely improve survival and health status and reduce hospitalizations in this patient population.

ACKNOWLEDGMENTS

Dr Salisbury is funded, in part, by the American Heart Association-Pharmaceutical Roundtable Outcomes Research Fellowship Program. Dr Kosiborod is funded, in part, by the American Heart Association Pharmaceutical Roundtable career development award in implementation research.

REFERENCES

1. Lloyd-Jones D, Adams R, Carnethon M, et al. Heart disease and stroke statistics–2009 update: a report from the American Heart Association Statistics Committee and Stroke Statistics Subcommittee. Circulation 2009;119(3):e21–181.
2. Stewart AL, Greenfield S, Hays RD, et al. Functional status and well-being of patients with chronic conditions. Results from the Medical Outcomes Study. JAMA 1989;262(7):907–13.
3. Braunstein JB, Anderson GF, Gerstenblith G, et al. Noncardiac comorbidity increases preventable hospitalizations and mortality among Medicare beneficiaries with chronic heart failure. J Am Coll Cardiol 2003;42(7):1226–33.
4. Lang CC, Mancini DM. Non-cardiac comorbidities in chronic heart failure. Heart 2007;93(6):665–71.
5. Groenveld HF, Januzzi JL, Damman K, et al. Anemia and mortality in heart failure patients: a systematic review and meta-analysis. J Am Coll Cardiol 2008; 52(10):818–27.
6. Komajda M, Anker SD, Charlesworth A, et al. The impact of new onset anaemia on morbidity and mortality in chronic heart failure: results from COMET. Eur Heart J 2006;27(12):1440–6.
7. Anand IS, Kuskowski MA, Rector TS, et al. Anemia and change in hemoglobin over time related to mortality and morbidity in patients with chronic heart failure: results from Val-HeFT. Circulation 2005; 112(8):1121–7.
8. O'Meara E, Clayton T, McEntegart MB, et al. Clinical correlates and consequences of anemia in a broad spectrum of patients with heart failure: results of the Candesartan in Heart Failure: Assessment of

Reduction in Mortality and Morbidity (CHARM) Program. Circulation 2006;113(7):986–94.

9. Horwich TB, Fonarow GC, Hamilton MA, et al. Anemia is associated with worse symptoms, greater impairment in functional capacity and a significant increase in mortality in patients with advanced heart failure. J Am Coll Cardiol 2002;39(11):1780–6.

10. Adams KF Jr, Pina IL, Ghali JK, et al. Prospective evaluation of the association between hemoglobin concentration and quality of life in patients with heart failure. Am Heart J 2009;158(6):965–71.

11. Al-Ahmad A, Rand WM, Manjunath G, et al. Reduced kidney function and anemia as risk factors for mortality in patients with left ventricular dysfunction. J Am Coll Cardiol 2001;38(4):955–62.

12. Komajda M. Prevalence of anemia in patients with chronic heart failure and their clinical characteristics. J Card Fail 2004;10(1 Suppl):S1–4.

13. Vasu S, Kelly P, Lawson WE. Anemia in heart failure– a concise review. Clin Cardiol 2005;28(10):454–8.

14. Tang YD, Katz SD. The prevalence of anemia in chronic heart failure and its impact on the clinical outcomes. Heart Fail Rev 2008;13(4):387–92.

15. Anand IS. Anemia and chronic heart failure implications and treatment options. J Am Coll Cardiol 2008; 52(7):501–11.

16. Kosiborod M, Curtis JP, Wang Y, et al. Anemia and outcomes in patients with heart failure: a study from the National Heart Care Project. Arch Intern Med 2005;165(19):2237–44.

17. Felker GM, Shaw LK, Stough WG, et al. Anemia in patients with heart failure and preserved systolic function. Am Heart J 2006;151(2):457–62.

18. Blanc B, Finch CA, Hallberg L. Nutritional anemias. Report of a WHO Scientific Group. World Health Organ Tech Rep Ser 1968;405:1–40.

19. Ishani A, Weinhandl E, Zhao Z, et al. Angiotensin-converting enzyme inhibitor as a risk factor for the development of anemia, and the impact of incident anemia on mortality in patients with left ventricular dysfunction. J Am Coll Cardiol 2005;45(3):391–9.

20. Adams KF Jr, Patterson JH, Oren RM, et al. Prospective assessment of the occurrence of anemia in patients with heart failure: results from the Study of Anemia in a Heart Failure Population (STAMINA-HFP) Registry. Am Heart J 2009;157(5):926–32.

21. Go AS, Yang J, Ackerson LM, et al. Hemoglobin level, chronic kidney disease, and the risks of death and hospitalization in adults with chronic heart failure: the Anemia in Chronic Heart Failure: Outcomes and Resource Utilization (ANCHOR) Study. Circulation 2006;113(23):2713–23.

22. Beutler E, Waalen J. The definition of anemia: what is the lower limit of normal of the blood hemoglobin concentration? Blood 2006;107(5):1747–50.

23. Ezekowitz JA, McAlister FA, Armstrong PW. Anemia is common in heart failure and is associated with

poor outcomes: insights from a cohort of 12,065 patients with new-onset heart failure. Circulation 2003;107(2):223–5.

24. Sharma R, Francis DP, Pitt B, et al. Haemoglobin predicts survival in patients with chronic heart failure: a substudy of the ELITE II trial. Eur Heart J 2004;25(12):1021–8.

25. Kosiborod M, Smith GL, Radford MJ, et al. The prognostic importance of anemia in patients with heart failure. Am J Med 2003;114(2):112–9.

26. Anand I, McMurray JJ, Whitmore J, et al. Anemia and its relationship to clinical outcome in heart failure. Circulation 2004;110(2):149–54.

27. Tang YD, Katz SD. Anemia in chronic heart failure: prevalence, etiology, clinical correlates, and treatment options. Circulation 2006;113(20):2454–61.

28. Anand IS, Chandrashekhar Y, Ferrari R, et al. Pathogenesis of oedema in chronic severe anaemia: studies of body water and sodium, renal function, haemodynamic variables, and plasma hormones [comment]. Br Heart J 1993;70(4):357–62.

29. Schrier RW, Abraham WT. Hormones and hemodynamics in heart failure. N Engl J Med 1999;341(8): 577–85.

30. McClellan WM, Flanders WD, Langston RD, et al. Anemia and renal insufficiency are independent risk factors for death among patients with congestive heart failure admitted to community hospitals: a population-based study. J Am Soc Nephrol 2002; 13(7):1928–36.

31. Kalra PR, Collier T, Cowie MR, et al. Haemoglobin concentration and prognosis in new cases of heart failure. Lancet 2003;362(9379):211–2.

32. Maraldi C, Volpato S, Cesari M, et al. Anemia, physical disability, and survival in older patients with heart failure. J Card Fail 2006;12(7):533–9.

33. Tang WH, Tong W, Jain A, et al. Evaluation and long-term prognosis of new-onset, transient, and persistent anemia in ambulatory patients with chronic heart failure. J Am Coll Cardiol 2008;51(5):569–76.

34. Peterson PN, Magid DJ, Lyons EE, et al. Association of longitudinal measures of hemoglobin and outcomes after hospitalization for heart failure. Am Heart J 2010;159:81–9.

35. Krumholz HM, Merrill AR, Schone EM, et al. Patterns of hospital performance in acute myocardial infarction and heart failure 30-day mortality and readmission. Circ Cardiovasc Qual Outcomes 2009;2(5):7.

36. Young JB, Abraham WT, Albert NM, et al. Relation of low hemoglobin and anemia to morbidity and mortality in patients hospitalized with heart failure (insight from the OPTIMIZE-HF registry). Am J Cardiol 2008;101(2):223–30.

37. Soto GE, Jones P, Weintraub WS, et al. Prognostic value of health status in patients with heart failure after acute myocardial infarction. Circulation 2004; 110(5):546–51.

38. Kosiborod M, Soto GE, Jones PG, et al. Identifying heart failure patients at high risk for near-term cardiovascular events with serial health status assessments. Circulation 2007;115(15):1975–81.

39. Spertus JA, Jones PG, Kim J, et al. Validity, reliability, and responsiveness of the Kansas City Cardiomyopathy Questionnaire in anemic heart failure patients. Qual Life Res 2008;17(2):291–8.

40. Kosiborod M, Krumholz HM, Jones PG, et al. The relationship between anemia, change in hematocrit over time and change in health status in patients with heart failure after myocardial infarction. J Card Fail 2008;14(1):27–34.

41. Nordyke RJ, Kim JJ, Goldberg GA, et al. Impact of anemia on hospitalization time, charges, and mortality in patients with heart failure. Value Health 2004;7(4):464–71.

42. Solid CA, Foley RN, Gilbertson DT, et al. Anemia and cost in Medicare patients with congestive heart failure. Congest Heart Fail 2006;12(6):302–6.

43. Allen LA, Anstrom KJ, Horton JR, et al. Relationship between anemia and health care costs in heart failure. J Card Fail 2009;15(10):843–9.

44. Felker GM, Gattis WA, Leimberger JD, et al. Usefulness of anemia as a predictor of death and rehospitalization in patients with decompensated heart failure. Am J Cardiol 2003;92(5):625–8.

45. Mozaffarian D, Nye R, Levy WC. Anemia predicts mortality in severe heart failure: the prospective randomized amlodipine survival evaluation (PRAISE). J Am Coll Cardiol 2003;41(11):1933–9.

46. Ezekowitz JA, McAlister FA, Armstrong PW. The interaction among sex, hemoglobin and outcomes in a specialty heart failure clinic. Can J Cardiol 2005;21(2):165–71.

47. Maggioni AP, Opasich C, Anand I, et al. Anemia in patients with heart failure: prevalence and prognostic role in a controlled trial and in clinical practice. J Card Fail 2005;11(2):91–8.

48. Valeur N, Nielsen OW, McMurray JJ, et al. Anaemia is an independent predictor of mortality in patients with left ventricular systolic dysfunction following acute myocardial infarction. Eur J Heart Fail 2006; 8(6):577–84.

49. Varadarajan P, Gandhi S, Sharma S, et al. Prognostic significance of hemoglobin level in patients with congestive heart failure and normal ejection fraction. Clin Cardiol 2006;29(10):444–9.

50. Dunlay SM, Weston SA, Redfield MM, et al. Anemia and heart failure: a community study. Am J Med 2008;121(8):726–32.

51. Kawashiro N, Kasanuki H, Ogawa H, et al. Clinical characteristics and outcome of hospitalized patients with congestive heart failure: results of the HIJC-HF registry. Circ J 2008;72(12):2015–20.

52. Anker SD, Voors A, Okonko D, et al. Prevalence, incidence, and prognostic value of anaemia in patients after an acute myocardial infarction: data from the OPTIMAAL trial. Eur Heart J 2009;30(11): 1331–9.

53. Hamaguchi S, Tsuchihashi-Makaya M, Kinugawa S, et al. Anemia is an independent predictor of long-term adverse outcomes in patients hospitalized with heart failure in Japan. A report from the Japanese Cardiac Registry of Heart Failure in Cardiology (JCARE-CARD). Circ J 2009;73(10):1901–8.

The Economic Burden of Anemia in Heart Failure

Richard K. Spence, MD, MHA[a,b],*

KEYWORDS

• Economic • Anemia • Heart failure • Quality of life

Anemia, although a seemingly simple diagnosis based on hemoglobin level (Hb), is a complex issue in patients with heart failure (HF). In past years, many clinicians accepted anemia as a given or an "accessory" diagnosis in HF patients in part because anemia was typically "mild" and effective treatment was not available. This attitude has changed since understanding of the causes and morbidity of anemia in HF has improved and with the introduction of targeted treatments, such as erythropoiesis-stimulating agents (ESA).

Moreover, increasing health care costs have stimulated vigorous debate about the cost-effectiveness of such treatments. Cost-effectiveness analysis compares the relative costs and outcomes or effects of 2 or more courses of action. Such analyses frequently use quality-adjusted life-years as a measure of the burden of the disease. Quality-adjusted life-years reflects the quality and quantity of life lived and is reported as the number of years added as a result of an intervention. It behooves clinicians to understand the effectiveness of specific treatments, their risks and benefits, and their costs to make reasoned and responsible decisions.

Many cost-effectiveness analyses in HF have been published on diverse topics, including New York Heart Association classification, type of medication, ventricular assist devices, and programmatic disease management approaches to treatment, but few have focused on anemia. This review addresses the impact of its prevalence, etiology, associated outcomes, and treatments on the economic burden in HF patients.

PREVALENCE

Many investigators have reported that anemia is common in patients with HF but the determination of actual prevalence is elusive, with reported ranges from 4% to more than 80%.[1–8] Prevalence varies depending on the time of presentation, the degree of HF, how anemia is defined, gender, presence or absence of renal failure, associated chronic illness, and the type of anemia. All play a role in how anemia is managed.

Time and disease progression influence the prevalence of anemia (**Table 1**). Reported incidence of new-onset anemia ranges from 15.9% to 53%.[7–12] Prevalence also increases over time—16% over 5 years in Dunlay and colleagues'[7,11] community study and 13% over 5 years in the Carvedilol or Metoprolol European Trial (COMET) trial. Although most reports use the World Health Organization definition for anemia—an Hb of less than 13 g/dL for men and less than 12 g/dL for women—some have used lower Hbs, which can skew prevalence calculations.[7,13] Tang and colleagues[14] reported that 17.2% of 6159 consecutive outpatients with CHF were anemic using lower Hbs of less than 12 g/dL for men and less than 11 g/dL for women. Half of the 48,612 patients included in the Organized Program to Initiate Lifesaving Treatment in Hospitalized Patients with

a Haemonetics, 400 Wood Road, Braintree, MA 02164, USA
b Robert Wood Johnson School of Medicine, University of Medicine and Dentistry of New Jersey, Davis Street and Copewood Avenue, Camden, NJ 08102, USA
* Corresponding address. 1828 Cardinal Lake Drive, Cherry Hill, NJ 08003.
E-mail address: rkspence@ix.netcom.com

Heart Failure Clin 6 (2010) 373–383
doi:10.1016/j.hfc.2010.02.003
1551-7136/10/$ – see front matter © 2010 Elsevier Inc. All rights reserved.

Table 1
Prevalence of anemia in HF patients

Author/Trial	Year	Patients (N)	% Anemic	Time of Onset
COMET[7]	2006	3029	15.9	New onset with 13% increase over time
Egelykke[9]	2006	163	23	New onset
Berry[10]	2006	528	45	New onset
Dunlay[11]—cohort 1	1979–2002	1063	40	New onset
Dunlay[11]—cohort 2	2003–2006	677	53	New onset with 16% increase over time
Choy[8]	2003–2006	170	47.6	New onset
Fabbri[12]	1995–2005	23,855	18.7	NA

Heart Failure (OPTIMIZE-HF) trial had low Hbs (12.1 g/dL); 25% had values of 5 to 10.7 g/dL.[15] It makes sense to use a standard World Health Organization definition of anemia in HF patients in future studies to avoid confusion.

HF patients often have coexistent renal failure, which increases the prevalence of anemia.[5,16,17] This combination of anemia, HF, and chronic kidney disease is frequently referred to as the cardiorenal anemia syndrome or cardiorenal syndrome (CRS).[16,18–23] Iania and associates[23] have characterized CRS as a vicious cycle of anemia that exacerbates chronic HF, thereby worsening the chronic renal failure, which in turn causes further anemia. Other chronic diseases, in particular hypertension and ischemic heart disease, are common in anemic HF patients.[24–26]

The author searched a database (COMPARE, Haemonetics, Braintree, Massachusetts, proprietary, unpublished data, 2007) of 883,257 inpatients admitted for a wide range of diagnoses to 20 hospitals from 2002 to 2007 to determine the prevalence of HF in this population. A total of 76,491 (8.7%) had a diagnosis of HF as determined by *International Classification of Diseases, Ninth Revision* codes. Of these, 16,916 (22%) had a principal diagnosis of HF. Patients had either left and right HF, 82.1% and 84.5%, respectively. The mean age was 68.2 ± 16.2 years; 52% were men and 48% were women; 40.5% were anemic on admission; and the mean admission Hb was 12.1 ± 0.03 SEM. More women were anemic on admission (women, 42%, and men, 38.5%) and more had a history of anemia (women, 21%, and men, 14%). Because 25% to 50% of HF patients develop anemia at some time during the course of their illness, physicians must be vigilant. At a minimum, this vigilance requires frequent measurements of Hb, hematocrit (Hct), iron status, and so forth, all of which add to the cost of treatment.

ETIOLOGY OF ANEMIA

Anemia in HF patients can be described as an "anemia of chronic disease" that is multifactorial. Several pathophysiologic interactions create a state of chronic immune-inflammatory activation with high levels of proinflammatory cytokines in cardiac tissues and the circulation.[27–30] Some cytokines interfere directly with renal tubular cell transcriptional messenger RNA activation by the EPO gene, thereby decreasing erythropoietin (EPO) production.[31–33] Others have been implicated as the cause of resistance of the bone marrow to EPO stimulation.[34,35] Cytokines also indirectly impair iron absorption, release, and use through generation of the protein hepcidin.[22,36,37]

Severe CRS involves a complex interactive network of cardiorenal connectors, which includes the renin-angiotensin system (RAS), nitric oxide, reactive oxygen species, the sympathetic nervous system, and inflammatory cytokines.[38–40] Interactions between angiotensin-converting enzyme (ACE) inhibitor therapy, the RAS, and anemia are of particular interest in this context.[29,41] van de Meer and colleagues[42] found in a group of 98 chronic HF patients that serum ACE levels were markedly lower in anemic patients and their sera inhibited erythropoietic progenitor cells from healthy patients. Terrovitis and colleagues[43] randomized 160 HF patients to standard (mean 17.9 ± 4.3 mg/d) or high (mean 42 ± 19.3 mg/d) doses of the ACE inhibitor, enalapril, and followed their prognosis for 2 years. Hct decreased significantly from 43.2 ± 4.9% at baseline to 40.7 ± 4.4% at 2 years (P<.001) in the high-dose group. β-Blocker therapy also may increase the risk of developing anemia, depending on the drug used. In the COMET study, treatment over 58 months with carvedilol versus metoprolol tartrate was associated with a 24% increased risk of developing new-onset anemia ($P = .0047$).[7]

Anemia in HF may be the result of iron deficiency, which can be caused by diet or chronic blood loss from the gastrointestinal tract, phlebotomy, dialysis, or cytokine-mediated functional iron deficiency. Iron deficiency anemia is often reported as one of the main causes of anemia in HF but few studies have reported prevalence.[44–47] Witte and colleagues[48] reported that "few" HF patients had iron deficiency in their comparative analysis of 296 patients and 58 control subjects of similar age. Nanas and colleagues[3] found deficient iron stores indicative of anemia in bone marrow aspirates from 27 of 37 (71%) HF patients.

Traditional methods of diagnosing anemia using volumetric tests of grams of Hb per deciliter or Hct measurement of percent of red blood cells (RBCs) per unit volume may need some refinement in HF patients because neither accounts adequately for the increased plasma volume in these patients. Adlbrecht and colleagues[46] studied 100 consecutive HF patients to determine the parameters associated with anemia. Their analysis included iron parameters, EPO and reticulocyte levels, hepcidin, glomerular filtration rate, plasma volume, and RBC volume. All factors played some role but hemodilution seemed the most significant predictor of low Hbs. They concluded that maintenance of renal function rather than just increasing RBC volume may help reduce the development of anemia in HF patients.

Patients with sickle cell disease, hereditary hemolytic anemia, or HIV-associated anemia may develop pulmonary hypertension, cor pulmonale, and HF.[49 51] An estimated 12% of patients with β-thalassemia develop HF as a consequence of their genetic defect and iron overload.[52,53] The most common anemia diagnosis in the author's COMPARE database patients was unspecified anemia (38.6%) followed by deficiency anemias (17.6%), acute blood loss anemia (16.5%), chronic anemia associated with end-stage renal disease (7.2%), hemolytic anemia (6.1%), and aplastic anemia (3.8%). The preponderance of unspecified anemia patients—more than one-third—suggests that clinicians need to pay more attention to identifying the cause of anemia in HF patients to promote focused treatment. Correct treatment of anemia demands an accurate diagnosis and focused treatment, both of which add to overall costs. Analysis of all the factors used by Adlbrecht and colleagues may be necessary to design appropriate therapy for anemia, which would lead to substantially increased diagnostic costs.

TREATMENT

It stands to reason that correction of underlying HF promotes a return to normal Hbs, given the pathophysiology (described previously).[54] Treatment of HF may have an opposite result, however. Reduction of plasma volume with diuretics increases Hct, seemingly correcting anemia, but RBC mass does not actually increase. Diuretics may also stimulate the renin-angiotensin system, which can lead to more fluid retention, vasoconstriction, and worsening HF.[55] β-Blockers may increase the risk of developing anemia in HF.[7] ACE inhibitors can worsen anemia through their effect on erythroid progenitor cells.[7,42,43] Furthermore, despite the use of ACE inhibitors, blockade of the RAAS may be incomplete, with continued production of angiotensin II by non–ACE-dependent pathways. Angiotensin receptor blockers have a proved benefit of reducing cardiac-related mortality in patients with impaired systolic function.[56] These drugs require close monitoring of the electrolytes, in particular serum potassium and renal function, adding to the cost of treatment. Although ACE and angiotensin receptor blocking drugs are relatively low cost, the need to tailor antihypertensive therapy to diminish the development of anemia may add to overall treatment costs.

The lack of consistency in HF treatment according to recommended guidelines makes it difficult to determine the magnitude of impact of treatment on overall costs and those associated with anemia. In the EPISERVE study, patients were treated by a variety of specialists and only 20% of patients received treatment recommended by clinical practice guidelines.[2] In 1999, Cleland and colleagues summarized mortality evidence from HF trials, warning that specialists tended to focus on treating comorbidities (eg, diabetes and not on HF).[57]

Correction of anemia with an ESA alone or in combination with intravenous iron is the generally accepted standard in patients with anemia of chronic disease. Results from several randomized trials comparing an ESA with oral iron and a placebo demonstrated that oral iron alone essentially has no effect.[58–62] Intravenous iron treatment has produced better results than oral iron and has led to significant improvement in left ventricular function, symptoms, and overall outcomes in HF patients.[45,47,63–67] ESA therapy, alone or in combination with intravenous iron, has produced the best results in correcting anemia in HF patients (**Table 2**).

Although most studies of ESA in HF patients have shown promising results, recent evidence from similar trials in anemic, non-HF patients has

Table 2
ESA treatment of anemia in heart failure patients: controlled randomized trials

Author	Year	Patients (N)	ESA	Iron	Time of Rx	Hgb (g/dL) PreRx	Hgb (g/dL) PostRx
Silverberg[97]	2006	32	rHuEPO	IV			
Kourea[61]	2008	41	Darbe 1.5 μg/kg daily	Oral	Every 20 days for 3 mo	10.9 ± 1.0	12.8 ± 1.4 g/dL
Mancini[98]	2003	26	15–30 Ku rHuEPO	No	Weekly	11.0 ± 0.5	14.3 ± 1.0
Palazzuoli[59]	2007	26	rHuEPO	Oral	Weekly for 4 mo	10.4 ± 0.6	12.4 ± 0.8
Cleland[99]	2005	33	Darbe 0.75 μg/kg, then 2, 3, or 5 μg/kg increase at second month	No	Monthly for 2 mo	≤12.5	2.3 ± 0.6, 1.4 ± 1.0, and 2.4 ± 1.9 g/dL, respectively, 4 wk after the second dose
van Veldhuisen[100]	2007	41	Darbe 0.75 μg/kg	No	Every 2 wk for 26 wk	9–12 g/dL	Increase of 1.5 g/dL
van Veldhuisen[100]	2007	1 = 56 2 = 55	1 = darbe weight adjusted 0.75 μg/kg 2 = darbe fixed dose 50 μg	No	27 wk	11.5 ± 0.7	1 = 13.4 2 = 13.2
STAMINA-HeFT[101]	2008	319	Titrated to target Hgb 14.0 g/dL	Oral	Every 2 wk for 1 y but measured at wk 27	11.4	Increase of 1.8 g/dL

Abbreviations: darbe, darbepoetin; Hgb, hemoglobin; IV, intravenous; Ku, kilounit; Rx, treatment.

raised concerns about an increased risk of morbidity and mortality from ESA treatment or high Hbs.[64,68] These concerns promoted the Correction of Hemoglobin and Outcomes in Renal Insufficiency (CHOIR) study group to do a post hoc analysis of their data.[69] In unadjusted analyses after 4 and 9 months, the inabilities to achieve a target Hb and high-dose recombinant human EPO (rHuEPO) were each significantly associated with increased risk of a primary endpoint (death, myocardial infarction [MI], congestive HF, or stroke). In adjusted models, high-dose rHuEPO was associated with a significantly increased hazard risk of reaching a primary endpoint but randomization to the high Hb was not. The investigators concluded that patients achieving their target Hb had better outcomes than those who did not and that there was no increased risk associated with the higher Hb. Iron and ESAs can correct anemia in HF patients, but they are often associated with higher, overall costs. As discussed previously, oral iron does not correct anemia in the majority of HF patients. Consequently, intravenous iron therapy, a more costly approach, is needed. ESA treatment with or without intravenous iron also corrects anemia but at an added cost. Choy and colleagues[8] reported that the costs associated with outpatient ESA and Iron therapy exceeded hospitalization cost savings by $83,070, concluding that a reduction in the cost of HFe-related hospitalization does not offset the cost of epoetin and intravenous iron therapy.

RBC transfusion, a standard treatment of anemia in HF, adds to hospital costs. The percentage of patients and the number of units transfused were greater in anemic compared with nonanemic CHF in the COMPARE database (Table 3). Anemic patients received 7368 units of RBCs compared with 2454 units in nonanemic patients, a difference of 4914 units. If this is multiplied by a typical cost of $500 for a transfusion episode, the increased cost of RBC transfusion in anemic CHF patients was $2,457,000.

ANEMIA, OUTCOMES AND COSTS

Anemia in HF patients significantly increases the risks of morbidity and mortality.[7,13,14,70–79] Iron deficiency anemia can worsen HF through left ventricular dilatation, with compensatory hypertrophy, which may progress to systolic dysfunction.[80,81] Anemic patients in the OPTIMIZE-HF registry had higher in-hospital mortality (4.8% vs 3.0%, lowest vs highest quartile), longer hospital LOS (6.5 vs 5.3 days), and more readmissions within 90 days after discharge (33.1% vs 24.2%; all $P<.0001$).[15] A prospective cohort design trial of the impact of anemia in 1130 HF patients conducted by Mozaffarian and colleagues[82] showed similar results. Over 15 months of mean follow-up, there were 407 deaths. After adjustment for potential confounders, those in the lowest quintile of Hct (range 25.4% to 37.5%) had a 52% higher risk of death (hazard ratio [HR] 1.52; 95% CI, 1.11 to 2.10), compared with the highest quintile (range 46.1% to 58.8%). Within the lowest quintile of Hct, each 1% decrease in Hct was associated with an 11% higher risk of death ($P<.01$).[83] Anemia was a significant predictor of a rapid decrease in renal function in 6360 HF patients enrolled in Studies of Left Ventricular Dysfunction (SOLVD).[84]

Groenveld and colleagues[85] reviewed 34 cohort and retrospective secondary analyses of randomized controlled trials of 153,180 HF patients to determine the impact of anemia on survival: 37.2% of the patients were anemic. After a minimal follow-up of 6 months, 46.8% of anemic patients died compared with 29.5% of nonanemic patients. Crude mortality risk of anemia was greater for anemic patients (OR 1.96; 95% CI, 1.74 to 2.21; $P<.001$). Adjusted HRs showed an increased risk for anemia (HR 1.46; 95% CI, 1.26 to 1.69; $P<.001$).

Data from the Centers for Medicare & Medicaid Services' National Heart Care Project that encompassed 50,405 patients 65 years and older discharged from acute care hospitals with a principal diagnosis of HF were subjected to multivariate logistic regression analyses by Kosiborod and colleagues[86] to determine if anemia was an independent predictor of mortality or readmission for HF-related events. Patients with an Hct less than or equal to 24% had a 51% higher relative risk (RR) of death (RR 1.51; CI, 1.35–1.68; $P<.001$) and a 17% higher risk of readmission (RR 1.17; CI, 1.01–1.34; $P<0.04$) compared with those whose Hcts were greater than 40% to 44%. The risk of mortality from anemia was less significant after adjustment for multiple comorbidities and clinical risk factors.

Table 3
Blood product use in anemic versus nonanemic congestive HF patients from COMPARE

Blood Product	Anemic Patients (N)	Nonanemic Patients (N)
RBC	2131	1014
Platelets	252	97
Fresh frozen plasma	483	249
Cryoprecipitate	31	19

Complications exact a great financial toll in HF patients: 1719 of 9531 (18%) of patients in the COMPARE database with a history of anemia developed complications compared with 4830 of 38,646 (12.5%) without anemia (P<.0001 for anemia). The development of a complication significantly increased total hospital charges as shown in **Table 4**. Charges were even greater in anemic patients.

Only a few investigators have reported directly on costs associated with anemia in congestive HF patients. Allen and colleagues[87] analyzed costs per year alive in 1056 patients with symptomatic HF seen at Duke University between 2002 and 2006. The adjusted costs per year alive for anemic patients were $22,926 compared with $17,189 for nonanemic patients (P = .04). Moreover, costs were higher still in patients with an ejection fraction of less than or equal to 40% ($32,914 for anemic vs $18,423 for nonanemic patients; P = .01). The Chronic Disease Research Group from Minnesota reported that the total cost to Medicare in 2003 to treat congestive HF patients with anemia was $1781.01 per member per month compared with $1142.38 for CHF patients without anemia. Costs remained 1.25 times higher after adjusting for baseline demographic factors and comorbid conditions.[88] Nissenson and colleagues[89] compared a private insurer's health resource use and costs for treatment of anemia in 118,332 patients who had chronic diseases with a randomized, control group of 35,948 similar nonanemic patients. This group included 14,985 anemic HF patients and 11,886 nonanemic HF patients. The average annualized health care payments per patient were significantly higher in anemic compared with nonanemic patients: $29,703 versus $12,459, respectively (P<.001). Payments attributed to treating anemia

alone were $1141 more than in nonanemic patients, a difference of 7%. Nordyke and colleagues'[90] retrospective analysis of claims data from October 1, 2000, to September 30, 2001, of 8569 HF patients addressed the economic impact of anemia in 3445 patients with an Hb of less than 12 g/dL. An increase in Hb of 1 g/dL was associated with a 5.1% reduction in LOS (P<.001) and a 4.3% decrease in charges (P<.001). The Institute for Advanced Studies in Aging and Geriatric Medicine conducted a similar, retrospective cohort study to estimate the differences in costs between anemic and nonanemic patients with chronic diseases that included HF.[91] Administrative claims data from 1999 through 2001 allowed them to assess direct costs, disability, and productivity data (1997–2001) to estimate indirect costs. The average annual direct costs were $72,078 for anemic HF patients, who incurred the greatest adjusted cost difference ($29,511) between anemic and nonanemic patients.

Studies that focus on the value of intravenous iron and ESA treatment in anemic HF patients show that this combined therapy is often effective in improving outcomes but is costly. Man-Fai Sim and colleagues[92] calculated the cost of anemia treatments in 86 elderly HF patients, then extrapolated costs to an estimated 1031 patients in their health district (total population 424,654). Cost of treatment with intravenous iron and ESA for the latter group was estimated at £7,000,000 per year. The investigators commented that the cost-effectiveness of this approach was unknown. As discussed previously in reference to Choy and colleagues,[8] outpatient ESA and iron therapy may not be cost-effective in reducing the cost of HF-related hospitalization. Silverberg and colleagues'[70] review of the impact

Table 4
Impact of complications on mean hospital charges in CHF patients with and without anemia

Variable	Charges with Complication	Charges Without Complication	Charges with Complication with Anemia	Charges with Complication Without Anemia	P Value for Both Comparisons
Clostridium difficile infection	$150,111	$54,822	$203,113	$62,189	<.0001
Acute MI	$71,753	$53,932	$94,140	$61,871	<.0001
Systemic Inflammatory Response Syndrome	$221,016	$52,598	$296,690	$59,128	<.0001
Postoperative Infection	$154,491	$54,202	$225,041	$61,693	<.0001
Pneumonia	$483,528	$57,667	$682,605	$69,514	<.0001
Pulmonary Complications	$500,843	$69,091	$734,475	$66,166	<.0001

of correction of anemia with ESAs and intravenous iron concluded that many studies showed reductions in number of hospitalizations, improvements in NYHA class, and quality of life but did not specifically address cost-effectiveness. Data clearly support the clinical benefit of combined intravenous iron and ESA treatment in anemic HF patients but the answer to the question of whether or not combined treatment is cost-effective remains elusive.

It is not only the presence of anemia but its persistence or duration that increases cost of treatment. The Chronic Disease Research Group from the University of Minnesota Twin Cities analyzed the impact of persistence of an Hb less than or equal to 11 g/dL, age, gender, treatment, and comorbidities, including HF, on economic outcomes in 28,985 incident dialysis patients.[93] Mean costs of treatment increased significantly with persistent anemia from $5461 at 0 months to $6276 at 1 to 2 months to $8070 at greater than or equal to 3 months. Costs were engendered by more EPO and RBC transfusions, more hospitalizations, more dialysis access procedures, and higher medical costs. In the 32.9% of patients with HF, 42.5% had persistent anemia and higher costs.

Anemia in general is associated with higher costs in hospitalized patients in part because length of stay (LOS) is often greater.[94,95] Anemic HF patients in the COMPARE database had significantly longer mean LOS when compared with nonanemic CHF patients (8.9 ± 0.1 SEM days vs 5.7 ± 0.1 SEM days, respectively; P<.0001). Mean total charges were significantly higher when compared with nonanemic patients ($46,883 ± 661 SEM vs $36,198 ± 579 SEM, respectively; P<.0001). Although it is difficult to calculate the mean cost for 1 day across a range of hospitals, the greater the number of days a patient is hospitalized, the greater the consumption of resources and the higher the cost. Increasing age, comorbidities (as determined by the Charlson index[96]), and female gender have been associated with increased costs in CHF patients and must be considered in any cost analysis.[88] The author found these same associations in the patient database; that is, all 3 variables were independently and statistically significant (P < .0001). Not all comorbidities have the same impact on charges and cost (as shown in **Table 5**). Several observations stand out: hospital charges for CHF patients without anemia are remarkably consistent within a few thousand dollars for all comorbidities; charges are higher in nonanemic patients with dementia, diabetes without sequelae, previous MI, cancer, and AIDS; and coexistent renal and hepatic failure are associated with a proportionally greater increase in charges than other comorbidities. All other variables remained significantly associated with increased charges after accounting for potential confounding. The overall model of variables

Table 5
Impact of comorbid conditions on mean hospital charges in CHF patients with and without anemia

Variable	Charges with Anemia	Charges without Anemia	P Value
Chronic renal failure	$81,353	$63.211	<.0001
Mild liver disease	$89,601	$64,415	<.0001
Connective tissue disease	$69,139	$69,368	0.15
Chronic obstructive pulmonary disease	$74,103	$62,615	<.0001
Cerebrovascular disease	$82,684	$63,942	<.0001
Peripheral vascular disease	$74,645	$64,096	<.0001
Dementia	$55,687	$68,065	<.0001
Diabetes mellitus	$62,129	$67,133	<.0001
Diabetic sequelae	$66,311	$65,514	0.52
Hemiplegia	$71,322	$67,503	0.05
Metastatic cancer	$72,518	$65,665	0.02
Previous MI	$61,017	$65,840	<.0001
Ulcer	$94,763	$67,085	<.0001
Cancer	$64,847	$66,526	0.17
AIDS	$56,435	$66,171	0.06
Severe liver disease	$136,373	$68,059	<.0001

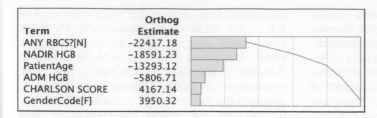

Term	Orthog Estimate	
ANY RBCS?[N]	−22417.18	
NADIR HGB	−18591.23	
PatientAge	−13293.12	
ADM HGB	−5806.71	
CHARLSON SCORE	4167.14	
GenderCode[F]	3950.32	

Fig. 1. Pareto plot of significant variables associated with charges in anemic CHF patients.

associated with charges did not change when presence of anemia on admission, actual Hb on admission, and lowest Hb during the hospitalization were added (for all, P <.0001). The addition of RBC transfusion, which was a univariable associated with increased cost, did not diminish the effect of comorbidities (**Fig. 1**). Moreover, a Pareto effect screening plot showed that RBC transfusion was the most important predictor of increased costs.

SUMMARY

This brief review of the economic impact of anemia in HF may have raised more questions than it has answered. The small number of detailed analyses of costs hampers knowledge, but the following is known.

Anemia in HF is common. Its cause is multifactorial, which mandates specific, more costly diagnostic and treatment approaches. Correction of anemia can improve clinical status in HF patients but treatment is expensive and the economic burden of treating anemic HF patients is significantly greater than that for nonanemic patients. This must be balanced by the knowledge that untreated anemia significantly increases the risk of morbidity and mortality in HF patients. More data are needed to determine which HF patients to treat and the type and duration of therapy to understand the cost-effectiveness of treatment of anemia.

REFERENCES

1. Mitchell JE. Emerging role of anemia in heart failure. Am J Cardiol 2007;99:15D–20D.
2. Gonzalez-Juanatey JR, Alegria Ezquerra E, Bertomeu Martinez V, et al. [Heart failure in outpatients: comorbidities and management by different specialists. The EPISERVE Study]. Rev Esp Cardiol 2008;61:611–9 [in Spanish].
3. Nanas JN, Matsouka C, Karageorgopoulos D, et al. Etiology of anemia in patients with advanced heart failure. J Am Coll Cardiol 2006;48:2485–9.
4. Grau-Amoros J, Formiga F, Jordana-Comajuncosa R, et al. [Anemia prevalence in heart failure. GESAIC study results]. Rev Clin Esp 2008;208:211–5 [in Spanish].
5. Stewart S, Wilkinson D, Hansen C, et al. Predominance of heart failure in the Heart of Soweto Study cohort: emerging challenges for urban African communities. Circulation 2008;118:2360–7.
6. Newton JD, Squire IB. Glucose and haemoglobin in the assessment of prognosis after first hospitalisation for heart failure. Heart 2006;92:1441–6.
7. Komajda M, Anker SD, Charlesworth A, et al. The impact of new onset anaemia on morbidity and mortality in chronic heart failure: results from COMET. Eur Heart J 2006;27:1440–6.
8. Choy CK, Spencer AP, Nappi JM. Prevalence of anemia in clinic patients with heart failure and cost analysis of epoetin treatment. Pharmacotherapy 2007;27:707–14.
9. Egelykke K, Petersen H, Haghfelt TH. [Prevalence and significance of anaemia in patients with chronic congestive heart failure]. Ugeskr Laeger 2006;168:1860–4 [in Danish].
10. Berry C, Norrie J, Hogg K, et al. The prevalence, nature, and importance of hematologic abnormalities in heart failure. Am Heart J 2006;151:1313–21.
11. Dunlay SM, Weston SA, Redfield MM, et al. Anemia and heart failure: a community study. Am J Med 2008;121:726–32.
12. Fabbri G, Gorini M, Maggioni AP, et al. [Italian Network on Congestive Heart Failure: ten-year experience]. G Ital Cardiol (Rome) 2006;7:689–94 [in Italian].
13. Dominguez Franco A, Pena Hernandez J, Perez Caravante M, et al. [Long-term prognosis value of anemia in a non-selected population with heart failure]. Med Clin (Barc) 2007;128:370–1 [in Spanish].
14. Tang WH, Tong W, Jain A, et al. Evaluation and long-term prognosis of new-onset, transient, and persistent anemia in ambulatory patients with chronic heart failure. J Am Coll Cardiol 2008;51:569–76.
15. Young JB, Abraham WT, Albert NM, et al. Relation of low hemoglobin and anemia to morbidity and mortality in patients hospitalized with heart failure (insight from the OPTIMIZE-HF registry). Am J Cardiol 2008;101:223–30.
16. Kazory A, Ross EA. Anemia: the point of convergence or divergence for kidney disease and heart failure? J Am Coll Cardiol 2009;53:639–47.
17. Lindenfeld J. Prevalence of anemia and effects on mortality in patients with heart failure. Am Heart J 2005;149:391–401.

18. Silverberg DS, Wexler D, Iaina A, et al. The interaction between heart failure and other heart diseases, renal failure, and anemia. Semin Nephrol 2006;26: 296–306.

19. Anand IS. Pathogenesis of anemia in cardiorenal disease. Rev Cardiovasc Med 2005;6(Suppl 3): S13–21.

20. McCullough PA, Lepor NE. The deadly triangle of anemia, renal insufficiency, and cardiovascular disease: implications for prognosis and treatment. Rev Cardiovasc Med 2005;6:1–10.

21. Cohen RS, Mubashir A, Wajahat R, et al. The cardio-renal-anemia syndrome in elderly subjects with heart failure and a normal ejection fraction: a comparison with heart failure and low ejection fraction. Congest Heart Fail 2006;12:186–91.

22. van der Putten K, Braam B, Jie KE, et al. Mechanisms of disease: erythropoietin resistance in patients with both heart and kidney failure. Nat Clin Pract Nephrol 2008;4:47–57.

23. Iaina A, Silverberg DS, Wexler D, et al. The cardio-renal anemia syndrome. Med Pregl 2007;60(Suppl 2): 145–50.

24. Sarmento PM, Fonseca C, Marques F, et al. Acutely decompensated heart failure: characteristics of hospitalized patients and opportunities to improve their care. Rev Port Cardiol 2006;25:13–27.

25. Maurer MS, Burkhoff D, Fried LP, et al. Ventricular structure and function in hypertensive participants with heart failure and a normal ejection fraction: the Cardiovascular Health Study. J Am Coll Cardiol 2007;49:972–81.

26. Tarmonova L, Shutov AM, Chernysheva EV. [Factors influencing left ventricular diastolic function in elderly patients with chronic heart failure]. Klin Med (Mosk) 2007;85:26–9 [in Russian].

27. Candia AM, Villacorta H Jr, Mesquita ET. Immune-inflammatory activation in heart failure. Arq Bras Cardiol 2007;89:183–90, 201–8.

28. Yndestad A, Damas JK, Oie E, et al. Systemic inflammation in heart failure—the whys and wherefores. Heart Fail Rev 2006;11:83–92.

29. Vasu S, Kelly P, Lawson WE. Anemia in heart failure—a concise review. Clin Cardiol 2005;28: 454–8.

30. Ferrucci L, Guralnik JM, Woodman RC, et al. Proinflammatory state and circulating erythropoietin in persons with and without anemia. Am J Med 2005;118:1288.

31. Stenvinkel P. The role of inflammation in the anaemia of end-stage renal disease. Nephrol Dial Transplant 2001;16(Suppl 7):36–40.

32. Macdougall IC, Cooper AC. Erythropoietin resistance: the role of inflammation and pro-inflammatory cytokines. Nephrol Dial Transplant 2002; 17(Suppl 11):39–43.

33. Means RT Jr. Recent developments in the anemia of chronic disease. Curr Hematol Rep 2003;2: 116–21.

34. Casadevall N. Cellular mechanism of resistance to erythropoietin. Nephrol Dial Transplant 1995; 10(Suppl 6):27–30.

35. Eisenstaedt R, Penninx BW, Woodman RC. Anemia in the elderly: current understanding and emerging concepts. Blood Rev 2006;20:213–26.

36. Matsumura I, Kanakura Y. [Pathogenesis of anemia of chronic disease]. Nippon Rinsho 2008;66:535–9 [in Japanese].

37. Opasich C, Cazzola M, Scelsi L, et al. Blunted erythropoietin production and defective iron supply for erythropoiesis as major causes of anaemia in patients with chronic heart failure. Eur Heart J 2005;26:2232–7.

38. Kes P, Basic-Jukic N, Juric I, et al. [The cardiorenal syndrome and erythropoietin]. Acta Med Croatica 2008;62(Suppl 1):21–31 [in Croatian].

39. Jie KE, Verhaar MC, Cramer MJ, et al. Erythropoietin and the cardiorenal syndrome: cellular mechanisms on the cardiorenal connectors. Am J Physiol Renal Physiol 2006;291:F932–44.

40. Perunicic-Pekovic G, Pljesa S, Rasic Z, et al. Relationship between inflammatory cytokines and cardiorenal anemia syndrome: treatment with recombinant human erythropoietin (rhepo). Hippokratia 2008;12:153–6.

41. Azizi M, Junot C, Ezan F, et al. Angiotensin I-converting enzyme and metabolism of the haematological peptide N-acetyl-seryl-aspartyl-lysyl-proline. Clin Exp Pharmacol Physiol 2001;28:1066–9.

42. van der Meer P, Lipsic E, Westenbrink BD, et al. Levels of hematopoiesis inhibitor N-acetyl-seryl-aspartyl-lysyl-proline partially explain the occurrence of anemia in heart failure. Circulation 2005; 112:1743–7.

43. Terrovitis JV, Anastasiou-Nana MI, Alexopoulos GP, et al. Prevalence and prognostic significance of anemia in patients with congestive heart failure treated with standard vs high doses of enalapril. J Heart Lung Transplant 2006;25:333–8.

44. van der Meer P, van Veldhuisen DJ. [New applications of erythropoietin in cardiovascular disease: from haematopoiesis to cardiac protection]. Ned Tijdschr Geneeskd 2008;152:923–7 [in Dutch].

45. Usmanov RI, Zueva EB, Silverberg DS, et al. Intravenous iron without erythropoietin for the treatment of iron deficiency anemia in patients with moderate to severe congestive heart failure and chronic kidney insufficiency. J Nephrol 2008;21:236–42.

46. Adlbrecht C, Kommata S, Hulsmann M, et al. Chronic heart failure leads to an expanded plasma volume and pseudoanaemia, but does not lead to

a reduction in the body's red cell volume. Eur Heart J 2008;29:2343–50.

47. Toblli JE, Lombrana A, Duarte P, et al. Intravenous iron reduces NT-pro-brain natriuretic peptide in anemic patients with chronic heart failure and renal insufficiency. J Am Coll Cardiol 2007;50:1657–65.

48. Witte KK, Desilva R, Chattopadhyay S, et al. Are hematinic deficiencies the cause of anemia in chronic heart failure? Am Heart J 2004;147:924–30.

49. Samuels-Reid JH. Common problems in sickle cell disease. Am Fam Physician 1994;49:1477–80, 83–6.

50. Gacon PH, Donatien Y. [Cardiac manifestations of sickle cell anemia]. Presse Med 2001;30:841–5 [in French].

51. Barnett CF, Hsue PY, Machado RF. Pulmonary hypertension: an increasingly recognized complication of hereditary hemolytic anemias and HIV infection. JAMA 2008;299:324–31.

52. Fucharoen S, Ketvichit P, Pootrakul P, et al. Clinical manifestation of beta-thalassemia/hemoglobin E disease. J Pediatr Hematol Oncol 2000;22:552–7.

53. Aessopos A, Kati M, Tsironi M. Congestive heart failure and treatment in thalassemia major. Hemoglobin 2008;32:63–73.

54. Mak G, Murphy NF, McDonald K. Anemia in heart failure: to treat or not to treat? Curr Treat Options Cardiovasc Med 2008;10:455–64.

55. Bayliss J, Norell M, Canepa-Anson R, et al. Untreated heart failure: clinical and neuroendocrine effects of introducing diuretics. Br Heart J 1987;57:17–22.

56. Demers C, Mody A, Teo KK, et al. ACE inhibitors in heart failure: what more do we need to know? Am J Cardiovasc Drugs 2005;5:351–9.

57. Cleland JG, McGowan J, Clark A, et al. The evidence for beta blockers in heart failure. BMJ 1999;318:824–5.

58. Palazzuoli A, Silverberg D, Iovine F, et al. Erythropoietin improves anemia exercise tolerance and renal function and reduces B-type natriuretic peptide and hospitalization in patients with heart failure and anemia. Am Heart J 2006;152(1096): e9–15.

59. Palazzuoli A, Silverberg DS, Iovine F, et al. Effects of beta-erythropoietin treatment on left ventricular remodeling, systolic function, and B-type natriuretic peptide levels in patients with the cardiorenal anemia syndrome. Am Heart J 2007;154(645):e9–15.

60. Parissis JT, Kourea K, Panou F, et al. Effects of darbepoetin alpha on right and left ventricular systolic and diastolic function in anemic patients with chronic heart failure secondary to ischemic or idiopathic dilated cardiomyopathy. Am Heart J 2008; 155(751):e1–7.

61. Kourea K, Parissis JT, Farmakis D, et al. Effects of darbepoetin-alpha on plasma pro-inflammatory cytokines, anti-inflammatory cytokine interleukin-10 and soluble Fas/Fas ligand system in anemic patients with chronic heart failure. Atherosclerosis 2008;199:215–21.

62. Kourea K, Parissis JT, Farmakis D, et al. Effects of darbepoetin-alpha on quality of life and emotional stress in anemic patients with chronic heart failure. Eur J Cardiovasc Prev Rehabil 2008;15:365–9.

63. Okonko DO, Grzeslo A, Witkowski T, et al. Effect of intravenous iron sucrose on exercise tolerance in anemic and nonanemic patients with symptomatic chronic heart failure and iron deficiency FERRIC-HF: a randomized, controlled, observer-blinded trial. J Am Coll Cardiol 2008;51:103–12.

64. Howlett JG. Recognition and treatment of anemia in the setting of heart failure due to systolic left ventricular dysfunction. Expert Rev Cardiovasc Ther 2008;6:199–208.

65. Garty M, Shotan A, Gottlieb S, et al. The management, early and one year outcome in hospitalized patients with heart failure: a national Heart Failure Survey in Israel—HFSIS 2003. Isr Med Assoc J 2007;9:227–33.

66. Silverberg DS, Wexler D, Blum M, et al. Effect of correction of anemia with erythropoietin and intravenous iron in resistant heart failure in octogenarians. Isr Med Assoc J 2003;5:337–9.

67. Iaina A, Silverberg DS, Wexler D. Therapy insight: congestive heart failure, chronic kidney disease and anemia, the cardio-renal-anemia syndrome. Nat Clin Pract Cardiovasc Med 2005;2:95–100.

68. Anand IS. Anemia and chronic heart failure implications and treatment options. J Am Coll Cardiol 2008;52:501–11.

69. Szczech LA, Barnhart HX, Inrig JK, et al. Secondary analysis of the CHOIR trial epoetin-alpha dose and achieved hemoglobin outcomes. Kidney Int 2008;74:791–8.

70. Silverberg DS, Wexler D, Iaina A, et al. The role of correction of anaemia in patients with congestive heart failure: a short review. Eur J Heart Fail 2008; 10:819–23.

71. Ceresa M, Capomolla S, Pinna G, et al. Anemia in chronic heart failure patients: comparison between invasive and non-invasive prognostic markers. Monaldi Arch Chest Dis 2005;64:124–33.

72. Tehrani F, Phan A, Morrissey R, et al. The prognostic value of anemia in patients with diastolic heart failure. Tex Heart Inst J 2009;36:220–5.

73. Karaye KM, Sani MU. Factors associated with poor prognosis among patients admitted with heart failure in a Nigerian tertiary medical centre: a cross-sectional study. BMC Cardiovasc Disord 2008;8:16.

74. Latado AL, Passos LC, Darze ES, et al. Comparison of the effect of anemia on in-hospital mortality in patients with versus without preserved left ventricular ejection fraction. Am J Cardiol 2006;98:1631–4.

75. O'Meara E, Clayton T, McEntegart MB, et al. Clinical correlates and consequences of anemia in a broad spectrum of patients with heart failure: results of the Candesartan in Heart Failure: assessment of reduction in mortality and morbidity (CHARM) program. Circulation 2006;113:986–94.

76. Felker GM, Shaw LK, Stough WG, et al. Anemia in patients with heart failure and preserved systolic function. Am Heart J 2006;151:457–62.

77. Sharma R, Francis DP, Pitt B, et al. Haemoglobin predicts survival in patients with chronic heart failure: a substudy of the ELITE II trial. Eur Heart J 2004;25:1021–8.

78. Varadarajan P, Gandhi S, Sharma S, et al. Prognostic significance of hemoglobin level in patients with congestive heart failure and normal ejection fraction. Clin Cardiol 2006;29:444–9.

79. Anand I, McMurray JJ, Whitmore J, et al. Anemia and its relationship to clinical outcome in heart failure. Circulation 2004;110:149–54.

80. O'Riordan E, Foley RN. Effects of anaemia on cardiovascular status. Nephrol Dial Transplant 2000;15(Suppl 3):19–22.

81. Clark SF. Iron deficiency anemia. Nutr Clin Pract 2008;23.120–41.

82. Mozaffarian D, Nye R, Levy WC. Anemia predicts mortality in severe heart failure: the prospective randomized amlodipine survival evaluation (PRAISE). J Am Coll Cardiol 2003;41:1933–9.

83. Szachniewicz J, Petruk-Kowalczyk J, Majda J, et al. Anaemia is an independent predictor of poor outcome in patients with chronic heart failure. Int J Cardiol 2003;90:303–8.

84. Bansal N, Tighiouart H, Weiner D, et al. Anemia as a risk factor for kidney function decline in individuals with heart failure. Am J Cardiol 2007;99:1137–42.

85. Groenveld HF, Januzzi JL, Damman K, et al. Anemia and mortality in heart failure patients a systematic review and meta-analysis. J Am Coll Cardiol 2008;52:818–27.

86. Kosiborod M, Curtis JP, Wang Y, et al. Anemia and outcomes in patients with heart failure: a study from the National Heart Care Project. Arch Intern Med 2005;165:2237–44.

87. Allen LA, Anstrom K, Horton J, et al. Relationship between anemia and health care costs in heart failure. J Card Fail 2009;15:639–726.

88. Solid CA, Foley RN, Gilbertson DT, et al. Anemia and cost in Medicare patients with congestive heart failure. Congest Heart Fail 2006;12:302–6.

89. Nissenson AR, Wade S, Goodnough T, et al. Economic burden of anemia in an insured population. J Manag Care Pharm 2005;11:565–74.

90. Nordyke RJ, Kim JJ, Goldberg GA, et al. Impact of anemia on hospitalization time, charges, and mortality in patients with heart failure. Value Health 2004;7:464–71.

91. Ershler WB, Chen K, Reyes EB, et al. Economic burden of patients with anemia in selected diseases. Value Health 2005;8:629–38.

92. Man-Fai Sim V, Nam MC, Riley S, et al. Anaemia in older people with chronic heart failure: the potential cost. Technol Health Care 2009;17:377–85.

93. The association of persistently low hemoglobin levels with medical expenditures in dialysis patients. Available at: http://www.cdrg.org/pub_pres/files/2006/15R_asn_06_low_hgb_costs.pdf. 2006. Accessed January 4, 2010.

94. Spence RK. Medical and economic impact of anemia in hospitalized patients. Am J Health Syst Pharm 2007;64:S3–10.

95. Ferraris VA, Ferraris SP. Risk factors for postoperative morbidity. J Thorac Cardiovasc Surg 1996;111:731–8 [discussion: 8–41].

96. Charlson M, Pompei P, Ales K, et al. A new method of classifying prognostic comorbidity in longitudinal studies: development and validation. J Chronic Dis 1987;40:373–83.

97. Silverberg DS, Wexler D, Sheps D, et al. The effect of correction of mild anemia in severe, resistant congestive heart failure using subcutaneous erythropoietin and intravenous iron: a randomized controlled study. J Am Coll Cardiol 2001;37:1775–80.

98. Mancini DM, Kunavarapu C. Effect of erythropoietin on exercise capacity in anemic patients with advanced heart failure. Kidney Int Suppl 2003;S48–52.

99. Cleland JG, Sullivan JT, Ball S, et al. Once-monthly administration of darbepoetin alfa for the treatment of patients with chronic heart failure and anemia: a pharmacokinetic and pharmacodynamic investigation. J Cardiovasc Pharmacol 2005;46:155–61.

100. van Veldhuisen DJ, Dickstein K, Cohen-Solal A, et al. Randomized, double-blind, placebo-controlled study to evaluate the effect of two dosing regimens of darbepoetin alfa in patients with heart failure and anaemia. Eur Heart J 2007;28:2208–16.

101. Ghali JK, Anand IS, Abraham WT, et al. Randomized double-blind trial of darbepoetin alfa in patients with symptomatic heart failure and anemia. Circulation 2008;117:526–35.

Future Directions in Management of Anemia in Heart Failure

Anil K. Agarwal, MD[a],*, Stuart D. Katz, MD[b]

KEYWORDS

- Anemia • Heart failure • Treatment • Therapy

Anemia is prevalent in patients with heart failure (HF) and progresses with worsening of cardiac function.[1] Multiple mechanisms including hemodilution, iron deficiency, or chronic kidney disease (CKD) have been attributed as causes of anemia.[2] Frequent presence of kidney disease in patients with HF also contributes to the development of anemia by causing erythropoietin deficiency.[3] Anemia, in turn, has been implicated In the pathophysiology of HF. There is a complex interaction between HF, renal failure, and anemia that often results in a vicious cycle known as cardiorenal anemia syndrome.[4] Aggravation of any of these conditions can result in the worsening of the other 2 conditions. Erythropoietin levels are known to be moderately elevated in HF, but these levels may be inadequate given the degree of anemia. Consequently, the treatment of anemia using erythropoiesis stimulating agents (ESAs) is hypothesized to lead to an improvement in various outcomes, including survival, exercise capacity, regression of left ventricular hypertrophy, reduction in NYHA (New York Heart Association) class and hospitalizations, and retardation of kidney disease progression. The results from a plethora of investigations show a striking variety of outcomes depending on patient population, presence or absence of kidney disease, and size (small or large) and design (noncontrolled or controlled) of the study. Future research in therapy of anemia in HF must take all these variables into consideration.

CURRENT EVIDENCE IN TREATMENT OF ANEMIA

Results of treatment of anemia in HF with ESAs have shown encouraging results. An uncontrolled study of correction of anemia in HF showed amelioration of symptoms, improvement in cardiac function, and reduction in hospitalizations.[5] Randomized controlled trials (RCTs) in HF have shown similar results. However, most studies of anemia correction in HF have used iron and ESA concurrently, making it difficult to interpret the individual effect of ESA or iron. Two studies using iron alone in HF have also shown salutary results.[6,7] Larger studies of iron and ESA in anemia and HF will help in defining their respective roles, benefits, and risks in patients with HF.

Coexistence of kidney disease with anemia and HF, not an uncommon occurrence, is associated with worse outcomes than those associated with either condition alone. The outcomes seem to be worsened by overzealous correction of anemia. Although cardiovascular (CV) outcomes of treatment of CKD anemia, such as left ventricular hypertrophy and CV events have been subjects of numerous studies, the guidelines for treatment of anemia in CKD do not specifically direct the

[a] Division of Nephrology, The Ohio State University, 395 West 12th Avenue, Ground Floor, Columbus, OH 43210, USA
[b] Division of Cardiology, School of Medicine, NYU Langone Medical Center, New York University, Skirball 9R, 550 First Avenue, New York, NY 10016, USA
* Corresponding author.
E-mail address: anil.agarwal@osumc.edu

Heart Failure Clin 6 (2010) 385–395
doi:10.1016/j.hfc.2010.03.004
1551-7136/10/$ – see front matter © 2010 Elsevier Inc. All rights reserved.

treatment of patients with associated heart disease because there are no specific and extensive studies of this subgroup. The Normal Hematocrit Study enrolled patients with end-stage renal disease (ESRD) with anemia receiving epoetin who had documented HF or ischemic heart disease in the previous 2 years.[8] In this study, 1233 anemic patients with ESRD were randomized to either partial correction of anemia to a 'low' hematocrit value of 32 or complete correction to a 'normal' hematocrit value of 42 of anemia using epoetin alfa. There were 99 patients with NYHA class I to III in the normal hematocrit group, and 98 in the low hematocrit group. Patients with NYHA class IV were excluded. After 29 months of follow-up, there was a 30% higher risk of primary outcome (death or nonfatal myocardial infarction [MI]) in the high-hematocrit group. Although this result was statistically nonsignificant, the study was discontinued because a high hematocrit value was not likely to improve outcomes. The mortality rate in each group actually decreased with a rise in hematocrit value. A recent post hoc analysis of the data has shown that a lower mortality rate was associated with a better relationship of epoetin dose with hematocrit response, although confounding by indication may be present (Fig. 1).[9,10]

THERAPEUTIC DILEMMA IN TREATMENT OF ANEMIA

Inconsistencies, controversies, and lack of information are the hurdles in the treatment of anemia. For example, treatment with ESA in patients with HF has been associated with improved outcomes, although the erythropoietin levels are elevated. The outcomes of treatment of anemia in patients with HF are encouraging, but it is not clear if the benefit is from iron or ESA. On the contrary, large RCTs of ESA for treatment of anemia in kidney disease have shown neutral or harmful effects when higher hemoglobin levels were targeted.[11,12] Mortality, strokes, progression or resurgence of cancer, and marginal improvement in quality of life have curbed the enthusiasm for treatment of CKD anemia with or without cardiac disease using ESA.[13] At present, there are no clearly defined targets of hemoglobin in CKD anemia, although a hemoglobin level of 10 g/dL seems to be a widely adopted goal. A 2007 revision of KDOQI guidelines recommended target hemoglobin range of 11 to 12 g/dL for all stages of CKD.[14] However, the Food and Drug Administration (FDA) recommends a more conservative target hemoglobin level of 10 to 12 g/dL for patients with CKD. Only the Caring For Australasians with Renal Impairment (CARI) guidelines from Australia have distinguished a distinct higher hemoglobin goal for patients with cardiovascular disease (CVD) revised guidelines now recommend an upper limit hemoglobin level of 13 g/dL, which is still a liberal goal considering the results of recent studies.[15] An even higher risk seems to be associated with treatment of anemia with ESA in patients with cancer.[16–18] Data from multiple studies in cancer have led the FDA to impose severe restrictions on the use of ESA in patients with cancer.

SAFETY OF LONG-TERM ESA THERAPY

The trend in use of ESA is currently in a state of flux, largely a result of recent RCTs showing adverse outcomes with high hemoglobin targets. Global safety data for ESA use are available from numerous observational and randomized controlled studies.

Since the initial uncontrolled observations reported by Silverberg and colleagues[19] spurred interest in the potential clinical benefits of ESA in anemic patients with HF, several investigator-initiated and industry-initiated randomized

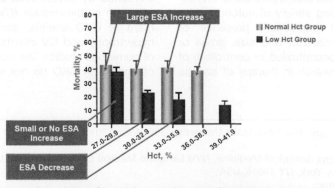

Fig. 1. ESA dose response and it relationship with mortality. Hct, hematocrit. (*From* Singh AK. The controversy surrounding hemoglobin and erythropoiesis-stimulating agents: what should we do now? Am J Kidney Dis 2008;52(S1):S5–13; with permission.)

clinical trials with recombinant erythropoietin preparations and darbepoetin alfa have been reported and summarized in a recent meta-analysis.[20] These investigators identified 7 randomized clinical trials that enrolled 650 subjects with HF and anemia (363 treated with erythropoiesis stimulating proteins and 287 control subjects). The largely concordant entry criteria for these studies were HF and systolic dysfunction with moderate anemia (average pretreatment hemoglobin level ranged from 10.3 g/dL to 11.8 g/dL) and without severe CKD (average serum creatinine levels ranged from 1.3 mg/dL to 2.2 mg/dL). The major finding of the meta-analysis was that the treatment with ESA was associated with a significant reduction in the risk for hospitalization (relative risk, 0.59; 95% confidence interval, 0.41–0.86, $P = .006$). There were few mortality events, and they did not differ between treatment groups (20 events in 363 subjects treated with ESA [5.5%] vs 25 events in 287 control subjects [8.7%], $P = .21$). Hypertension and venous thrombosis occurred at low rates, with no difference between treatment groups. In a small number of subjects, Mancini and colleagues[21] demonstrated that erythropoietin treatment that targeted a hemoglobin level of 14.5 g/dL did not alter regional vascular resistance in the forearm at rest or in response to transient ischemia and did not alter blood pressure at rest or during exercise. A pooled analysis of the adverse effect profile of darbepoetin alfa in anemic patients with HF confirms these findings.[22] The 3 studies in this pooled analysis (all sponsored by Amgen, Inc, Thousand Oaks, CA, USA) included 516 of the 650 subjects in the meta-analysis and provided much greater detail on the clinical characteristics of the study population and the rates of adverse events independently adjudicated according to prespecified criteria by a panel blinded to study treatment assignment. Hemoglobin levels increased significantly in subjects treated with darbepoetin alfa (0.50–0.75 µg/kg every 2 weeks) when compared with placebo (mean change from baseline to 6 months was 1.9 g/dL in darbepoetin alfa group vs 0.5 g/dL in placebo group, $P<.001$). There were no differences between groups for all reported adverse events (darbepoetin alfa 87% vs placebo 85%), treatment-related adverse events (darbepoetin alfa 12% vs placebo 9%), adverse events requiring withdrawal from study treatment (darbepoetin alfa 3% vs placebo 4%), or all reported serious adverse events (darbepoetin alfa 37% vs placebo 43%). The rates of serious adverse events, including hypertension, worsening HF, MI, stroke or transient ischemic attack, deep vein thrombosis, and pulmonary emboli, did not differ between treatment groups.

Although the total number of anemic subjects with HF in published clinical trials is small, preliminary data indicate that the safety profile of ESA in the population with HF may differ from that observed in the populations with CKD and cancer. One factor that may reduce the risk of thromboembolic events in the population with HF is the common use of antiplatelet medications (65%) and oral anticoagulation (25%).[22] The use of supplemental iron in these trials is also different from that in CKD populations. Most of the subjects in HF trials were treated with oral but not intravenous supplemental iron. Despite negligible use of intravenous iron, there were minimal changes in measures of iron stores in the darbepoetin alfa group (serum ferritin decreased 11 ± 11 ng/mL from pretreatment value of 177 ± 196 ng/mL; serum iron increased 1.7 ± 0.8 µmol/L from pretreatment value of 14.2 ± 6.1 µmol/L; and transferrin saturation decreased 2.7% ± 1.2% from baseline value of 26.7% ± 10.6%). These findings are not unexpected because patients with clinically evident iron deficiency were excluded from the study, and the small increment in hemoglobin levels in response to darbepoetin therapy (1.5–2.0 gm/dL) was not likely to exhaust normal iron stores. Finally, the entry criteria for all but one of the HF clinical trials excluded patients with comorbid severe CKD. It is possible that other unmeasured confounding clinical variables present in anemic patients with CKD and cancer, but not in patients with HF, may contribute to the different safety profile.

The known limitations of meta-analysis and other forms of pooled analysis limit the translation of the existing studies into clinical practice decision making. The Reduction of Events with darbepoetin alfa in Heart Failure (RED-HF, Clinical Trials.gov NCT 003 58215) study is an industry-sponsored, international double-blind randomized trial to determine the effects of darbepoetin alfa (doses ranging from 20 to 600 µg subcutaneously every 2–4 weeks to achieve target hemoglobin of 13 g/dL) versus matching placebo on a combined primary end point of all-cause mortality and hospitalization in anemic patients with HF and systolic dysfunction.[23] Key entry criteria include hemoglobin level of 9 to 12 g/dL and left ventricular ejection fraction of 40% or less. Key exclusion criteria include poorly controlled hypertension, serum creatinine level greater than 3.0 mg/dL, and transferrin saturation less than 15%. Supplemental iron (oral or intravenous) will be administered if transferrin saturation decreases to less than 20% during the course of the study. The trial is event-driven, expected to enroll 2600 subjects over a 4- to 5-year period, and is to be completed in 2012. The results of this study should provide definitive data on the safety and efficacy of treatment with an ESA in anemic patients with HF.

Several RCTs have been conducted in CKD arena to examine the role of ESA therapy on CV outcomes and quality of life. Most of the studies had a significant number of patients with preexisting CVD, making the results relevant to cardiologists and nephrologists. Important results of the studies of anemia treatment in patients with ESRD or nondialysis CKD are summarized in **Tables 1** and **2**, respectively.

It is important to examine the safety data from 2 large RCTs published in 2006. The Correction of Hemoglobin and Outcomes in Renal Insufficiency (CHOIR) trial enrolled 1432 patients in the United States to study the risks of anemia correction using epoetin.[11] The patients were randomized to subcutaneous epoetin alfa to achieve hemoglobin level of either 13.5g/dL (n = 715) or 11.3g/dL (n = 717). Median study duration was 16 months. There were a significantly higher number of primary composite end points (death, MI, hospitalization for congestive HF, and stroke) in the high-hemoglobin group. It was concluded that a high hemoglobin target was associated with an increased mortality risk and no incremental improvement in quality of life . ESA dose was higher in the high-target group. Patients not achieving their target in either group received higher doses of epoetin and had similar risks of adverse outcomes. The study was limited by an open-label design, high dropout rate (38%), and the actual achieved mean hemoglobin level of 12.6 g/dL despite higher doses of epoetin. Nonetheless, the study demonstrated elevated risk of high hemoglobin target in patients with CKD anemia. The Cardiovascular Risk Reduction by Early Anemia Treatment with Epoetin Beta (CREATE) study was a randomized, controlled, multinational trial that enrolled 603 anemic patients with CKD stage 3 to 4 to achieve target hemoglobin level of 13 to 15 g/dL with epoetin beta in group 1 and to maintain 10.5 to 11.5 g/dL in group 2.[12] The study did not find significant difference in primary end point of a composite of 8 CV events between the 2 groups. Decline in estimated glomerular filtration rate (GFR) was similar, although dialysis was required in more patients in group 1. General health and physical function

improved in group 1. The study was limited by a smaller annual event rate (6%) than expected (15%). There was a 3 times higher annual event rate in the CHOIR study, indicating a more severe CV risk in that population. In both studies, the group having higher hemoglobin levels received higher doses of iron. The epoetin dose was much higher in CHOIR study compared with the dose in CREATE study.

The recently published Trial to Reduce Cardiovascular Events with Aranesp Therapy (TREAT) enrolled patients with CKD (estimated GFR, 20–60 mL/min) with type 2 diabetes and anemia (hemoglobin<11gm/dL).[13] In contrast to other trials comparing high and low hemoglobin targets, this multicenter, double-blind, placebo-controlled trial randomized 4038 patients to either treatment with darbepoetin alfa to raise hemoglobin level to 13 g/dL or treatment with placebo (unless the hemoglobin level dipped to <9 g/dL when rescue treatment with darbepoetin alfa was provided). Approximately two-thirds of the patients in each group had a history of CVD. The primary end points of composite outcomes of death or a CV event (nonfatal MI, congestive HF, stroke, or hospitalization for myocardial ischemia) and of death or ESRD were not different between the 2 groups after a median follow-up of 29.1 months. There was an increased risk for stroke in the active treatment group, but the transfusions were significantly more in the placebo group. The results of this study suggest caution in treating diabetic patients with CKD and anemia using ESA because of a heightened risk for stroke.

FUTURE DIRECTIONS FOR THERAPY OF ANEMIA

The selection of the optimal end points for clinical trials in patients with HF is complicated by the complex nature of the disease process, the difficulty in interpretation of surrogate end-point changes, and the regulatory environment for drug development. One approach used successfully in the African-American Heart Failure Trial (A-HeFT) is the incorporation of a composite score using surrogate measures of disease severity (exercise testing, quality-of-life questionnaires, and/or global assessments) that are relevant to the anticipated physiologic effects of the agent under investigation, in combination with the occurrence of morbidity and mortality events.[29] In the case of ESA, intravenous iron, and other agents intended to effect an increase in hemoglobin levels, some assessment of maximal exercise tolerance is a reasonable surrogate end point to include within a composite score.

Table 1
Published RCTs of treatment of anemia in patients on dialysis

Study	Number	Population	Target Hemoglobin (g/dL) vs Hematocrit	Design	Primary Outcome	Follow-up (mo)	Cardiovascular Outcome	Quality of Life
Besarab et al[8]	1233	HD-CHF/CAD	30 vs 42	Open label	Death, MI	29	No difference	Improved
Foley[24]	146	HD-CHF/CAD	9.5–10.5 vs 13–14	Open label	LVMI, LVVI	12	No difference	Improved
Parfrey[25]	596	HD-CHF/CAD	9.5–11.5 vs 13.5–?	Double blind	LVVI	22	No difference	Improved

Abbreviations: CAD, coronary artery disease; CHF, congestive heart failure; HD, heart disease; LVMI, left ventricular mass index; LVVI, left ventricular volume index.
Data from a Robert Toto presentation, Current Controversies in Anemia: Current KDOQI Recommendations—Target hemoglobin levels and CVD Risk, National Kidney Federation meeting, 2007.

Table 2
Published RCTs of treatment of anemia in patients with CKD not on dialysis

Study	Number	Population	Target Hemoglobin (g/dL) vs Hematocrit	Design	Primary Outcome	Follow-up (mo)	CV Outcome	Quality of Life
Roger[26]	155	Stage 3–5	9–10 vs 12–13	Open label	Δ LVMI	24	No difference	Improved
Levin[27]	172	Stage 2–5	9.0–10.5 vs 12–14	Open label	LVMI	22.6	No difference	Improved
Singh[11]	1432	Stage 4–5	11–11.5 vs 13–13.5	Open label	Death, CV event	16	Worse in high hemoglobin	No difference
Druecke[28]	603	Stage 4–5	11–11.5 vs 13–15	Open Label	Death, CV event	36	No difference	Improved

Abbreviations: LVMI, left ventricular mass index; Δ, change in LVMI.
Data from a Robert Toto presentation, Current Controversies in Anemia: Current KDOQI Recommendations—Target hemoglobin levels and CVD Risk, National Kidney Federation meeting, 2007.

EMERGING THERAPIES FOR ANEMIA

Epoetin alfa was the first ESA to be used primarily for anemia of CKD, later used for HF as well. Other epoetins, including epoetin beta, delta, and zeta, are in therapeutic use around the world. In the last decade, darbepoetin alfa was approved by FDA in the United States and had the advantage of longer half-life, making it possible to extend the dosing interval up to once a month. The continuous erythropoietin receptor activator is a pegylated recombinant human erythropoietin with an even longer half-life. It has been approved for use in renal anemia in the European Union. There has been search for other erythropoietic molecules. Hematide is an investigational synthetic pegylated erythropoietin mimetic peptide with a peptide sequence that is different from that of natural or recombinant erythropoietin. However, it stimulates erythropoietin receptor in the same manner as native or recombinant erythropoietin. The dissimilarity makes it suitable for the treatment of pure red cell aplasia occurring with epoetin or darbepoetin administration.[30] Hematide holds interesting future prospects in determining CV outcomes. Hypoxia inducible factor (HIF) 1 alpha stimulates production of erythropoietin in conditions of hypoxia but is degraded by prolyl hydroxylase (PH) inhibitors. A novel strategy to increase the native erythropoietin production is the use of stabilizers of HIFs that inhibit the PH activity. The oral PH inhibitors allow HIF-1 alpha stabilization despite normoxia and result in stimulation of erythropoiesis. These agents are currently under clinical trials.

The erythropoietin receptor is present in many nonerythropoietic tissues, including endothelium, vascular smooth muscle cells, myocardium, and neurons.[31,32] Preliminary data from pilot studies of short-term administration of ESA in patients with acute MI have demonstrated its safety, but data from 2 larger efficacy studies are yet to be reported.[33–35] As erythropoietin has shown tissue-protective properties because of its antiapoptotic action, it would be interesting to develop a selective ligand for this receptor with cytoprotective therapy but without erythropoiesis stimulation.

IRON, ESA HYPORESPONSIVENESS, HEPCIDIN, AND INFLAMMATION

Iron deficiency is present in about one-third of HF cases. However, it is not always possible to accurately diagnose iron deficiency from anemia of chronic illness because of the acute phase nature of iron parameters.[36] A low-dose oral iron absorption test showing increment in iron levels after 2 hours of administration of 10 mg ferrous sulfate solution has been considered helpful in demonstrating the value of oral iron administration but is not commonly performed.[37] There is a correlation of anemia with high levels of proinflammatory cytokines, including tumor necrosis factor α (TNF-α), Interleukin (IL) 1, IL-6, and C-reactive protein, which cause a blunting of erythropoietin response to anemia. Hepcidin, secreted by the liver in response to IL-6, downregulates the expression of ferroportin thereby decreasing iron absorption from the duodenum. Thus, inflammation, via hepcidin can perpetuate iron deficiency and has to be considered as a target of anemia therapy.

ESA hyporesponsiveness remains a common problem in therapy for anemia. With evidence of harm from high ESA dose, it is worthwhile to investigate the possibility of decreasing ESA usage by recognizing and treating the factors related to ESA resistance. Iron deficiency is a common cause of poor ESA response, but the patients with HF may not respond to oral iron administration. Using ESA in presence of iron deficiency can also lead to thrombocytosis that can increase the risk of thrombosis.[38] To avoid adverse CV outcomes associated with high-dose ESA therapy, the use of iron may increase for treatment of anemia. Concerns in iron therapy include anaphylactic reactions (mostly with old preparations of iron dextran), oxidative stress, and free radical formation.

RESPONSE TO IRON THERAPY

Intravenous iron has been used in anemic patients with CKD and HF. A study of aggressive supplementation of intravenous iron in hemodialysis patients showed improvement in hemoglobin level and sparing of ESA.[39] Because of the inefficacy of oral iron in patients with HF, intravenous iron has been studied in this group of anemic patients. A small (n = 16), nonrandomized trial of intravenous iron (without ESA) showed improvement in hemoglobin and exercise capacity.[7] In the Ferric Iron Sucrose in Heart Failure (FERRIC-HF) study (n = 35), there was no significant difference in change in hemoglobin level in the treatment group compared with placebo, although there was improvement in ferritin level, functional class based on Patient Global Assessment, and NYHA functional class.[40] Another small (n = 40) placebo-controlled trial of intravenous iron in patients with HF and renal insufficiency showed reduction in NT-pro-brain natriuretic peptide in anemic patients.[6,41] A recent randomized, placebo-controlled trial (Ferinject assessment in patients with iron deficiency and chronic heart failure [Fair-HF]) of intravenous ferric carboxymaltose in patients (n = 459) with HF and iron deficiency, with or without anemia, showed improvement in symptoms, functional capacity, and quality of life in the treatment group.[40] The side-effect profile was acceptable. Patients are currently being recruited for a randomized trial to assess the effects of iron supplementation in patients with HF and anemia (Iron-HF).[42] Encouraging results from these studies, with improvement in cytokines, suggest that iron therapy alone may be preferred for treatment of anemia of HF, although large randomized controlled studies with attention to safety data will be necessary before such a recommendation is made.

HEMOGLOBIN VARIABILITY AND CV OUTCOMES

Hemoglobin, like most other biologic variables, fluctuates in normal individuals, although the amplitude of this change is small. Under the influence of ESA stimulation, this variability is amplified in anemic individuals. The term "hemoglobin cycling" has been given to the cyclic variations in hemoglobin levels in patients with anemia of CKD. These variations occur in response to dose adjustments of iron and ESA to keep hemoglobin levels in a desired range over a period of time and can be tracked by the values obtained for hemoglobin monitoring. The fluctuations can also be a result of intercurrent illnesses, and wide swings in the hemoglobin levels perhaps indicate unstable clinical status. Although hemoglobin variability has been linked to higher mortality, such an interpretation of hemoglobin variability is fraught with a high degree of confusion.[43,44] In a recent study of patients on long-term hemodialysis (n = 159,720), patients with a hemoglobin level that fell to a low value or that showed variability at the low end of the hemoglobin range had the highest risk of mortality.[45] Although observational, the data from this large cohort of patients with ESRD substantiate the hypothesis that the association of variability with higher mortality is important to consider in sick patients with low hemoglobin who are likely to receive higher dosage of ESA and iron.

Variability of hemoglobin level in patients with HF may be partly attributed to changes in plasma volume in response to dietary sodium and diuretic therapy. Androne and colleagues[46] used a validated radiolabeled albumin technique to measure plasma volume and red blood cell volume in 37 anemic patients with HF. Nearly half of the patients (46%) had expanded plasma volume (hemodilution) as the cause of anemia because the red blood cell volume was in the normal range. Hemodilution was associated with increased pulmonary capillary wedge pressure and mortality risk when compared with patients with anemia and decreased red blood cell volume. These findings have been confirmed in subsequent studies that demonstrated that increased fluid retention (as determined by measurement of extracellular volume by a radiolabeled iothalamate technique) and increased plasma volume (determined by red blood cell chromium labeling) were the most powerful predictors of low hemoglobin levels in anemic patients with HF.[47,48] In contrast, Nanas and colleagues[36] demonstrated hemodilution (assessed by red blood cell chromium labeling) in only 5% of anemic patients with HF. The divergent findings might, in part, be related to patient selection and background therapy or to differences in techniques used to measure plasma volume.[49] Nonetheless, these studies indicate that at least some patients with HF have a low hematocrit value primarily because of plasma volume expansion. The optimum treatment strategy for patients with hemodilution as the primary cause of anemia has not been determined.

IMPACT OF NEW DATA ON PRACTICE

The recent evidence from multiple RCTs appropriately suggests caution in using ESA for treatment of anemia. However, the role of lower dosages of these agents to achieve lower targets, catered to the individual, is yet to be defined. Outside the setting of an RCT, several factors including comorbidities, hospitalizations, concomitant medications, and high mortality of this sick population may create confounding by indication and make interpretation of nonexperimental data difficult.[50] It is unlikely that the optimal dose of ESA, hemoglobin target, and iron parameters will ever be defined in an individual, and the art of medicine will be needed to fill the void in the absence of such evidence. Simultaneously, early evidence of benefits of iron therapy will lead to increasing use of intravenous iron, although more evidence of benefits and safety are needed from larger trials.

Blood transfusions are frequently needed for those with symptomatic anemia with HF. Transfusions are well known to be associated with significant risks, including infection, allosensitization, and iron overload. The supply of units of red cells is limited, and any increase in number of packed red blood cells because of the changes in anemia management strategy may be highly consequential. The threshold for transfusion is not well established in patients with HF, which is largely individualized according to the presence or absence of symptoms. In a study of elderly patients with acute MI, transfusion to keep the hematocrit value greater than 30% was associated with survival benefit.[51] However, use of transfusions to achieve this level on a consistent basis does not seem to be a preferred approach. With cautious use of ESA in CKD, which is a co-morbid condition in almost 40% of the patients with HF, it is likely that the transfusion requirements will increase.

The explosion in academic investigation and exponential increase in the acquisition of knowledge relevant to the pathogenesis and potential treatment options have clearly identified anemia as an important clinical factor to consider in HF and have provided novel insight into the complex pathophysiology of HF, but some important questions are still unanswered, such as the optimal means to evaluate the cause of anemia in clinical settings and identification of patients most likely to derive clinical benefit from treatment. Ongoing studies with ESA and intravenous iron preparations in the population with HF and with novel agents in other anemic populations may provide important data for clinical decision making over the next few years. Meanwhile, the risk benefit analysis must be evaluated for each patient, with treatment decisions based on extrapolation from limited data in the population with HF and National Kidney Foundation consensus guidelines for the subpopulation of patients with HF with anemia and concomitant CKD.

REFERENCES

1. Anand IS. Anemia and chronic heart failure. Implications and treatment options. J Am Coll Cardiol 2008; 52:501–11.
2. Tang Y, Katz SD. Anemia in chronic heart failure: Prevalence, etiology, clinical correlates, and treatment options. Circulation 2006;113:2454–61.
3. McClellan WM, Flanders WD, Langston RD, et al. Anemia and renal insufficiency are independent risk factors for death among patients with congestive heart failure admitted to community hospitals: a population-based study. J Am Soc Nephrol 2002; 13:1928–36.
4. Silverberg DS, Wexler D, Iaina A, et al. The interaction between HF and other heart diseases, renal failure, and anemia. Semin Nephrol 2006; 26:296–306.
5. Silverberg DS, Wexler D, Blum M, et al. The interaction between heart failure, renal failure and anemia-the cardio-renal anemia syndrome. Kidney Blood Press Res 2005;28:41–7.
6. Toblli JE, Lombraña A, Duarte P, et al. Intravenous iron reduces NT-pro-brain natriuretic peptide in anemic patients with chronic heart failure and renal insufficiency. J Am Coll Cardiol 2007;50:1657–65.
7. Bolger AP, Bartlett FR, Penston HS, et al. Intravenous iron alone for the treatment of anemia in patients with chronic heart failure. J Am Coll Cardiol 2006;48:1225–7.
8. Besarab A, Bolton WK, Browne JK, et al. The effects of normal as compared with low hematocrit values in patients with cardiac disease who are receiving hemodialysis and epoetin. N Engl J Med 1998;339: 584–90.
9. Kilpatrick RD, Critchlow CW, Fishbane S, et al. Greater epoetin alfa responsiveness is associated with improved survival in hemodialysis patients. Clin J Am Soc Nephrol 2008;3:1077–83.
10. Singh AK. The controversy surrounding hemoglobin and erythropoiesis-stimulating agents: what should we do now? Am J Kidney Dis 2008;52(S1):S5–13.
11. Singh AK, Szczech L, Tang KL, et al. Correction of anemia with epoetin alfa in chronic kidney disease. N Engl J Med 2006;355:2085–98.
12. Drueke TB, Locatelli F, Clyne N, et al. Normalization of hemoglobin level in patients with chronic kidney disease and anemia. N Engl J Med 2006;355: 2071–84.
13. Pfeffer MA, Burdmann EA, Chen C-Y, et al. A trial of darbepoetin alfa in type 2 diabetes and chronic kidney disease. N Engl J Med 2009;361:2019–32.
14. National Kidney Foundation KDOQI. KDOQI clinical practice guideline and clinical practice recommendations for anemia in chronic kidney disease: 2007 update of hemoglobin target. Am J Kidney Dis 2007;50:471–530.
15. Available at: http://www.cari.org.au/DIALYSIS_bht_published/Haemoglobin_Aug_2008.pdf. Accessed January 24, 2010.
16. Wun T, Law L, Harvey D, et al. Increased incidence of symptomatic venous thrombosis in patients with cervical carcinoma treated with concurrent chemotherapy, radiation, and erythropoietin. Cancer 2003;98:1514–20.
17. Henke M, Laszig R, Rube C, et al. Erythropoietin to treat head and neck cancer patients with anaemia undergoing radiotherapy: randomised, double-blind, placebo-controlled trial. Lancet 2003;362:1255–60.
18. Leyland-Jones B, Semiglazov V, Pawlicki M, et al. Maintaining normal hemoglobin levels with epoetin alfa in mainly nonanemic patients with metastatic breast cancer receiving first-line chemotherapy: a survival study. J Clin Oncol 2005;23:5960–72.
19. Silverberg DS, Wexler D, Blum M, et al. The use of subcutaneous erythropoietin and intravenous iron for the treatment of the anemia of severe, resistant congestive heart failure improves cardiac and renal function and functional cardiac class, and markedly reduces hospitalizations. J Am Coll Cardiol 2000;35: 1737–44.
20. van der Meer P, Groenveld HF, Januzzi JL, et al. Erythropoietin treatment in patients with chronic heart failure: a meta-analysis. Heart 2009;95: 1309–14.

21. Mancini DM, Katz SD, Lang CC, et al. Effect of eryth-ropoietin on exercise capacity in patients with moderate to severe chronic heart failure. Circulation 2003;107:294–9.

22. Klapholz M, Abraham WT, Ghali JK. The safety and tolerability of darbepoetin alfa in patients with anaemia and symptomatic heart failure. Eur J Heart Fail 2009;11:1071–7.

23. McMurray JJ, Anand IS, Diaz R, et al. Design of the reduction of events with darbepoetin alfa in heart failure (RED-HF): a Phase III, anaemia correction, morbidity–mortality trial. Eur J Heart Fail 2009;11: 795–801.

24. Foley RN, Parfrey PS, Morgan J, et al. Effect of hemo-globin levels in hemodialysis patients with asymptom-atic cardiomyopathy. Kidney Int 2000;58:1325–35.

25. Parfrey PS, Foley RN, Wittreich BH, et al. Double-blind comparison of full and partial correction in incident hemodialysis patients without symptomatic heart disease. J Am Soc Nephrol 2005;16:2180–9.

26. Roger SD, McMahon LP, Clarkson A, et al. Effects of early and late intervention with epoetin alpha on left ventricular mass among patients with chronic kidney disease (stage 3 or 4): results of a randomized clinical trial. J Am Soc Nephrol 2004;15:148–56.

27. Drueke T, Eckardt K, Scherhag A. Correspondence. N Engl J Med 2007;356(9):959.

28. Levin A, Djurdjev O, Thompson C, et al. Canadian randomized trial of hemoglobin maintenance to prevent or delay left ventricular mass growth in patients with CKD. Am J Kidney Dis 2005;46: 799–811.

29. Franciosa JA, Taylor AL, Cohn JN, et al. African-Amer-ican Heart Failure Trial (A-HeFT): rationale, design and methodology. J Card Fail 2002;8:128–35.

30. Macdougall IC, Rossert J, Casadevall N, et al. A peptide-based erythropoietin-receptor agonist for pure red-cell aplasia. N Engl J Med 2009;361: 1848–55.

31. Wu H, Lee SH, Gao J, et al. Inactivation of erythro-poietin leads to defects in cardiac morphogenesis. Development 1999;126:3597–605.

32. Cerami A, Brines M, Ghezzi P, et al. Neuroprotective properties of epoetin alfa. Nephrol Dial Transplant 2002;17(Suppl 1):8–12.

33. Lipsic E, van der Meer P, Voors AA, et al. A single bolus of a long-acting erythropoietin analogue dar-bepoetin alfa in patients with acute myocardial infarction: a randomized feasibility and safety study. Cardiovasc Drugs Ther 2006;20:135–41.

34. Liem A, van de Woestijne AP, Bruijns E, et al. Effect of EPO administration on myocardial infarct size in patients with non-STE acute coronary syndromes; results from a pilot study. Int J Cardiol 2009;131: 285–7.

35. Tang Yi-da, Hasan F, Giordano F, et al. Effects of recombinant human erythropoietin on platelet activation in acute myocardial infarction: results of a double-blind, placebo-controlled, randomized trial. Am Heart J 2009;158:941–7.

36. Nanas JN, Matsouka C, Karageorgopoulos D, et al. Etiology of anemia in patients with advanced heart failure. J Am Coll Cardiol 2006;48:2485–9.

37. Jensen NM, Brandsborg M, Boesen AM, et al. Low-dose oral iron absorption test in anaemic patients with and without iron deficiency determined by bone marrow iron content. Eur J Haematol 1999; 63:103–11.

38. Beguin Y, Loo M, R'Zik S, et al. Effect of recombinant human erythropoietin on platelets in patients with anemia of renal failure: Correlation of platelet count with erythropoietic activity and iron parameters. Eur J Haematol 1994;53:265–70.

39. Coyne DW, Kapoian T, Suki W, et al. Ferric gluconate is highly efficacious in anemic hemodialysis patients with high serum ferritin and low transferrin satura-tion: Results of the Dialysis Patients' Response to IV Iron with elevated ferritin (DRIVE) study. J Am Soc Nephrol 2007;18:975–84.

40. Anker SD, Colet JC, Filippatos G, et al. Ferric car-boxymaltose in patients with heart failure and iron deficiency. N Engl J Med 2009;361:2436–48.

41. Francis GS, Kanderian A. Anemia and heart failure. A new pathway. J Am Coll Cardiol 2007; 50:1666–7.

42. Beck-da-Silva L, Rohde LE, Periera-Barretto AC, et al. Rationale and design of the IRON-HF study: a randomized trial to assess the effects of iron supplementation alone on the functional capacity in heart failure patients with anemia. J Card Fail 2007;13:14–7.

43. Ebben JP, Gilbertson DT, Foley RN, et al. Hemo-globin level variability: associations with comorbidity intercurrent events, and hospitalizations. Clin J Am Soc Nephrol 2006;1:1205–10.

44. Brunelli SM, Joffe MM, Israni RK, et al. History adjusted marginal structural analysis of the associa-tion between hemoglobin variability and mortality among chronic hemodialysis patients. Clin J Am Soc Nephrol 2008;3:777–82.

45. Gilbertson DT, Ebben JP, Foley RN, et al. Hemo-globin level variability: associations with mortality. Clin J Am Soc Nephrol 2008;3:133–8.

46. Androne AS, Katz SD, Lund L, et al. Hemodilution is common in patients with advanced heart failure. Circulation 2003;107:226–9.

47. Westenbrink BD, Visser FW, Voors AA, et al. Anaemia in chronic heart failure is not only related to impaired renal perfusion and blunted erythropoi-etin production, but to fluid retention as well. Eur Heart J 2007;28:166–71.

48. Adlbrecht C, Kommata S, Hülsmann M, et al. Chronic heart failure leads to an expanded plasma volume and pseudoanaemia, but does not lead to

a reduction in the body's red cell volume. Eur Heart J 2008;29:2343–50.

49. Katz SD. Blood volume assessment in the diagnosis and treatment of chronic heart failure. Am J Med Sci 2007;334:47–52.

50. Bradbury BD, Brookhart MA, Winkelmayer WC, et al. Evolving statistical methods to facilitate evaluation of the causal association between erythropoiesis stimulating agent dose and mortality in nonexperimental research: strengths and limitations. Am J Kidney Dis 2009;54:554–60.

51. Wu WC, Rathore SS, Wang Y, et al. Blood transfusion in elderly patients with acute myocardial infarction. N Engl J Med 2001;345:1230–6.

Index

Note: Page numbers of article titles are in **boldface** type.

A

Anemia, and iron stores, 300–301
  bio-similars in, 353
  cardiorenal, multidisciplinary approach to, xi–xvi
  definition of, 271
  emerging therapies for, 391
  erythropoietin receptor activator in, 353
  etiology of, 290–292, 374–375
  GATA inhibitors in, 353–354
  hemopoietic cell phosphatase in, 354
  hospital performance measures and, 368
  hypoxia-inducible factor stabilizers in, 354
  in chronic heart failure, 306
    age as factor in, 289
    chronic kidney disease and, 290
    clinical characteristics associated with, 289–290
    erythropoietin production and, 291–292
    female gender and, 289–290
    functional capacity and fluid retention in, 290
    iron metabolism and, 290–291
    mediators of, **289–293**
    pathogenesis of, 295
    renin-angiotensin system and, 292
    structural and molecular changes in, 295–296
  in chronic kidney disease, correction of, erythropoietin-stimulating agents and, 327–330
    erythropoietin-stimulating agents and iron in, adverse events due to, 352–353
    high mortality in, 327–330
    new advances in, **347–357**
  in heart failure, and renin-angiotensin system, 282
    causes and confounders of, 273–276
    causes of, 279–282, 326
    chronic inflammation and, 276
    cost of care in, 370
    demographic data and, 275
    diabetes mellitus and, 275
    disease severity and, 274–275
    drug therapy in, impact of, 276–277
    economic burden of, **373–383**
    epidemiology of, **271–278**
    health status outcomes of, 368–370
    hematologic data and, 271–272
    hemodilution and, 276, 282
    hospitalization and, 368
    in chronic kidney disease, 279, 284
      and impaired erythropoietin production, 280–282
    in hematinic abnormalities, 279–280
    incidence of, 273, 274
    management of, future directions in, **385–395**
    mechanisms of, 281
    morbidity and mortality associated with, 276
    mortality associated with, 365–367
    outcomes and costs associated with, 377–380
    outcomes associated with, **359–372**
    oxygen delivery in, hemodynamic mechanisms to maintain, 283
      non-hemodynamic mechanisms maintaining, 282–283
    pathophysiological consequences of, 282
    pathophysiology of, **279–288**
    poor outcomes in, explanation of, 283–284
    preserved versus impaired ejection fraction and, 275
    prevalence of, 272–273, 359–365, 373–374
    profile of patients with, 279
    red blood cell transfusion in, 377
    renal insufficiency and, 275
    treatment of, 375–377
      blood transfusions in, 392–393
      current evidence in, 385–386
      erythropoiesis-stimulating agents in, 385, 386
      therapeutic dilemma in, 386
  in patients not on dialysis, treatment of, trials on, 390
  in patients on dialysis, treatment of, trials on, 389
  iron deficiency, in chronic heart failure, 307
  mortality in heart failure with or without, 366
  of chronic disease, 282, 295
  or iron deficiency, molecular changes in myocardium in, **295–304**
  renal outcomes in, 323–326
  treatment of, newer molecules for, 353–354

B

Bio-similars, in anemia, 353
Blood transfusions, in anemia in heart failure, 392–393
Bone marrow endothelial progenitor cells, and erythropoietin signaling, 298

C

Cardiorenal anemia, multidisciplinary approach to, xi–xvi

Heart Failure Clin 6 (2010) 397–399
doi:10.1016/S1551-7136(10)00060-7
1551-7136/10/$ – see front matter © 2010 Elsevier Inc. All rights reserved.

Cardiorenal syndrome(s), acute, epidemiology of, 336–337
    acute management of, 337–340
    chronic, epidemiology of, 335–336
    classification of, definitions of, and work group statements on, xiv–xv
    end of life care in, 341
    epidemiology of, **333–346**
    longitudinal care in, 340–341
    mortality due to, 341
       increased, explanations for, 337
    pathophysiology and risk factors for, 333–335
    subtypes of, xii–xiii
    types of, 333, 334

D

Death, risk of, heart failure and hematocrit related to, 323, 324
Diabetes mellitus, and anemia in heart failure, 275
Dialysis, anemia in patients on, treatment of, trials of, 389
Disease, chronic, anemia of, 295

E

Endothelial progenitor cells, bone marrow, and erythropoietin signaling, 298
Epoetin alfa, in anemia, 353
Erythropoiesis-stimulating agents, and iron, in anemia and chronic kidney disease, adverse events due to, 352–353
    hyporesponsiveness to, 391
    in chronic kidney disease, 324–326
       cardiovascular outcomes of, 327
    in heart failure, cardiovascular outcomes in, 326–327
    in treatment of anemia in heart failure, 385, 386
    long-term therapy using, safety of, 386–388
    therapy with, renal and nonrenal outcomes of, **323–332**
Erythropoiesis stimulation, in acute ischemic syndromes, **313–321**
Erythropoietin, and ischemia, clinical studies of, 316–318
    as cytoprotective agent, studies of, 316–318
    biologic functions of, 313, 314
    cardioprotective signaling by, 296
    cytoprotection and, 315
    production of, 296, 313
       and anemia in chronic heart failure, 291–292
       impaired, and anemia in heart failure, 280–282
       in chronic heart failure, 296
    recombinant, 313, 351
    signaling, improved, myocardial changes due to, 297–298

synthesis and effects of, 296, 297
Erythropoietin-erythropoietin function receptor system, and ischemia, animal studies in, 313–316
Erythropoietin function receptor, 315
Erythropoietin receptor, modulation of, 351
Erythropoietin receptor activator, in anemia, 353

F

Ferric Iron Sucrose in Heart Failure trial, 308–309
Fluid retention, in anemia in chronic heart failure, 290

G

GATA inhibitors, in anemia, 353–354

H

Heart failure, and hematocrit, related to risk of death, 323, 324
    anemia in. See *Anemia, in heart failure*.
    chronic, erythropoietin production in, 296
       iron stores in, 298–299
    mortality in, with and without anemia, studies of, 366
    parenteral supplementation of iron in, 308–310
    symptoms of, iron deficiency and, 307–308
    with and without anemia, treatment with iron, **305–312**
Hematinic abnormalities, anemia in heart failure in, 280–282
Hematocrit, heart failure and, related to risk of death, 323, 324
Hematologic data, and anemia in heart failure, 271–272
Hemodilution, and anemia in heart failure, 276, 282–283
Hemoglobin, levels of, change in, over time, and mortality, 367
    variability of, and cardiovascular outcomes, 392
Hemoglobin-oxygen dissociation curve, 282–283
Hemoglobin target level, evolving, 351–352
Hemopoietic cell phosphatase, in anemia, 354
Hepcidin, in chronic kidney disease, 349–350
    iron absorption and, 391
    iron regulation and, 300, 349
Hospital performance measures, anemia and, 368
Hospitalization, and anemia in heart failure, 368
Hypoxia-inducible factor stabilizers, in anemia, 354

I

Intestine, in iron homeostatis, 348–349
Iron, absorption of, hepcidin and, 391
    and erythropoiesis-stimulating agents, in anemia and chronic kidney disease, adverse events due to, 352–353

distribution of, in adults, 348
metabolism of, and anemia in chronic heart failure,
   290–291
   proteins in, 300
regulation of, hepcidin and, 300, 349
storage of, assessment of, 306
   physiology of, 305–306
supplementation of, parenteral, in heart failure,
   308–310
treatment with, in heart failure with and without
   anemia, **305–312**
   response to, in chronic kidney disease,
      391–392
Iron deficiency, and symptoms of heart failure,
   307–308
   in chronic heart failure, 306–307
   management of, advances in, 350–351
   or anemia, molecular changes in myocardium in,
      295–304
Iron homeostasis, in chronic kidney disease, 347–350
   intestine and liver in, 348–349
   kidney in, 349
Iron stores, anemia and, 300–301
   in chronic heart failure, 298–299
   myocardial changes due to, 299–301
Ischemia, erythropoietin and, clinical studies of,
   316–318
Ischemic syndromes, acute, erythropoiesis
   stimulation in, **313–321**

K

Kidney disease, chronic, and anemia in chronic heart
   failure, 290
      and anemia in heart failure, 279, 284
      and impaired erythropoietin production, and
         anemia in heart failure, 280–282
      erythropoiesis-stimulating agents in, 324–326
         cardiovascular outcomes of, 327
      hecipin in, 349–350

   iron homeostasis in, 347–350
      response to iron therapy in, 391–392
   dialysis in, treatment of anemia and, 390
Kidneys, conditions in, in anemia, 323–326
   in iron homeostasis, 349
   therapy with erythropoiesis-stimulating agents
      and, **323–332**

L

Liver, in iron homeostasis, 348–349

M

Myocardium, changes in, due to improved
   erythropoietin signaling, 297–298
      due to iron stores, 299–301
   molecular changes in, in anemia or iron deficiency,
      295–304

N

National Kidney Foundation/Disease Outcome
   Quality Initiative guideline, 350

R

Red blood cell transfusion, in anemia in heart failure,
   377
Renal insufficiency, and anemia in heart failure, 275
Renin-angiotensin system, and anemia in chronic
   heart failure, 292
   and anemia in heart failure, 282

T

Transfusions, in anemia in heart failure, 377, 392–392

Our issues help you manage *yours.*

NEW!

CARDIAC ELECTROPHYSIOLOGY CLINICS

Consulting Editors: Ranjan K. Thakur, MD, MPH, FHRS, and Andrea Natale, MD, FACC, FHRS

ISSN: 1877-9182 • Published Quarterly

www.cardiacep.theclinics.com

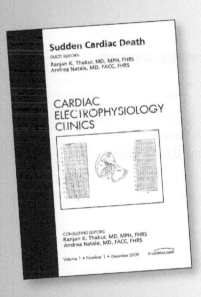

Four times a year,

Cardiac Electrophysiology Clinics...

- equips you with expert reviews on **the latest solutions** to problems you face every day.

- features hardbound and online issues that serve as **complete, succinct monographs** on specific topics relevant to your practice.

- presents guest editors and contributors who explore each topic from a **variety of perspectives**.

- delivers practical advice on **how to make the best use of the newest techniques and approaches.**

2010 Topics include:

Epicardial Interventions in Electrophysiology ■ Advances in Arrhythmia Analyses: A Case-Based Approach ■ Arrhythmogenic Right Ventricular Cardiomyopathy/Dysplasia ■ Advances in Antiarrhythmic Drug Therapy

Full-text online access to each issue as it publishes is included with your personal subscription

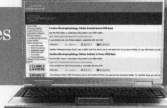

ELSEVIER

SUBSCRIBE TODAY!

1-800-654-2452 (U.S. and Canada) • **314-447-8871** (outside U.S. and Canada)

Visit **www.us.elsevierhealth.com/clinics**

Moving?

Make sure your subscription moves with you!

To notify us of your new address, find your **Clinics Account Number** (located on your mailing label above your name), and contact customer service at:

Email: journalscustomerservice-usa@elsevier.com

800-654-2452 (subscribers in the U.S. & Canada)
314-447-8871 (subscribers outside of the U.S. & Canada)

Fax number: 314-447-8029

**Elsevier Health Sciences Division
Subscription Customer Service
3251 Riverport Lane
Maryland Heights, MO 63043**

*To ensure uninterrupted delivery of your subscription, please notify us at least 4 weeks in advance of move.

Printed and bound by CPI Group (UK) Ltd, Croydon, CR0 4YY
03/10/2024
01040359-0014